HCG Diet Cookbook

Easy, Modern & Healthy Gourmet Recipes for Rapid Weight Loss (Contains 2 Texts: The HCG Diet Cookbook & The HCG Diet – A Step by Step Guide to Rapid Fat Loss)

The HCG Diet Cookbook

66 Easy Recipes for Rapid Fat Loss, Laser Sharp Focus and a Better Life (Lose up to a Pound a Day!)

the information in question by the reader will render any resulting actions solely under their purview. There are no scenarios in which the publisher or the original author of this work can be in any fashion deemed liable for any hardship or damages that may befall them after undertaking information described herein.

Additionally, the information found on the following pages is intended for informational purposes only and should thus be considered, universal. As befitting its nature, the information presented is without assurance regarding its continued validity or interim quality. Trademarks that are mentioned are done without written consent and can in no way be considered an endorsement from the trademark holder.

Table of Contents

Introduction

Congratulations on downloading your personal copy of *The HCG Diet Cookbook*. Thank you for doing so.

The following chapters will provide you with lots of HCG friendly recipes. Each recipe will state which phase of the diet it is most beneficial to so that you don't have to guess.

There are four phases of the HCG diet. The first phase in the loading phase and lasts the first two days. Here you will eat foods high in calories and fat. This is to prevent you from feeling as hungry during your first week. You will also start with you HCG supplements.

Phase two is the HCG phase and will last for 21 to 40 days. During this time you will weigh yourself each morning after using the bathroom. You will continue with the HCG, and you will eat a diet of 500 calories. This continues until you have lost the weight you want.

Phase three is the stabilization phase. Between phase two and phase three, you will have two days to transition where you stop taking HCG but continue the low-calorie diet. Once you enter stabilization, you will start consuming more calories and foods, but starches and sugars are not allowed. Your calories should stay between 1000 and 1500. This will last for 21 days.

Phase four is the maintenance phase and will continue for the rest of your life. You will continue a healthy diet and only indulge every now and then.

There are plenty of books on this subject on the market, thanks again for choosing this one! Every effort was made to ensure it is full of as much useful information as possible. Please enjoy!

Breakfast

Egg Baked Tomato

Servings: 4
Phase 3

Ingredients:
Pepper
Salt
1 tbsp. ghee
4 eggs
2 bacon slices, diced and cooked
4 ripe tomatoes

Directions:
Your oven should be at 425. Slice off the tops of all the tomatoes. With a fork, spoon or paring knife, clean the insides out of the tomatoes. You are basically making a tomato bowl.

Divide the cooked bacon between the four bowls. Beat each of the eggs separately and pour one into each of the four tomato bowls over the bacon.

Split the ghee between the tomatoes and place on top of the eggs. Season everything with some pepper and salt.

Place them in a baking dish and bake for 40-50 minutes.

Serve and Enjoy!

Granola

Servings: 4
Phase 4

Ingredients:
1/3 c raisins
1 tbsp. brown sugar
1 tsp. cinnamon
1 tsp. vanilla
1 tbsp. vegetable oil
1 tbsp. Stevia
2 tbsp. honey
¼ tsp. salt
Cooking spray
2 tbsp. chopped almonds
¼ c oat bran
2 tbsp. chopped walnuts
1 c oats

Directions:
Your oven should be at 300.

Combine together the nuts, oats, and oat bran. Place this to the side.

Take a cookie sheet and coat it with some cooking spray and set to the side.

In a little pot, mix together the vanilla, cinnamon, vegetable oil, honey, brown sugar, Stevia, and salt.

Heat it until it almost starts to boil. Stir every few minutes so that none of it clumps up. Set it off the heat and let it cool slightly.

Once it has cooled off, mix in the raisins,

Pour this over your oat mixture and stir it all together until well coated.

Spread this over your greased cookie sheet.

Set in the oven for 30 to 32 minutes.

Slice the granola into squares and keep stored in an air tight container.

Omelet

Servings: 1
Phase 3

Ingredients:
2 oz. meat – your choice
½ avocado
½ c shredded cheese – your choice
4 onions
2 tbsp. water
3 eggs
3 egg whites – you can use egg substitute

Directions:
Coat a skillet with some nonstick spray and let it heat up.

Mix together the onion, water, and all the eggs until well mixed. Pour the mixture into your hot pan.

When it starts to set up a bit, lift the sides with a spatula so that they raw egg on top runs under.

Sprinkle the omelet with cheese and place on a lid and cook for a couple of minutes.

Place on the avocados and meat, and any other healthy toppings you may want.

Fold the omelet in half and enjoy.

Vegetable Omelet

Servings: 1
Phase 3

Ingredients:

1 tbsp. parsley
2 oz. cheddar cheese, shredded
¼ tsp. salt
1 – 2 tsp. hot sauce
4 eggs
Nonstick spray
¼ c mushrooms, sliced
¼ c chopped bell pepper
¼ c onion, chopped
2 oz. cheddar cheese, shredded
1 small yellow squash, chopped
1 small tomato, chopped and seeded
1 small zucchini, chopped

Directions:

Lightly spray your skillet with nonstick spray then pour oil and let it heat up.

Mix together the salt, hot sauce, and eggs. Cook the egg mixture in the skillet.

When the eggs start to set, lift the eggs to allow the uncooked liquid to flow to the bottom.

Once the egg is cooked, top with cheese and veggies.

Place a lid on a let veggies steam for a bit.

Once done, fold in half and enjoy.

Greek Yogurt and Berries

Servings: 1
Phase 3

Ingredients:
1 tsp. fresh lemon juice
1 to 2 packets Stevia, powdered
¼ c raspberries
¼ c blueberries
¼ c strawberries
¾ c Greek yogurt, unsweetened and plain

Directions:
Slice up the strawberries and cut the raspberries in half if they are large. Place all of your berries into a serving bowl.

After squeezing the lemon juice, sprinkle Stevia over the berries. Stir everything together until fully mixed.

Cover the bowl and let it cool in the fridge for an hour. Stir the berries every 15 minutes. This will help to break the berries down and release juice.

Once the fruit is juicy, take them out and mix in the Greek yogurt. Add more Stevia if you need to, and enjoy.

Applesauce

Servings: 1
Phase 2

Ingredients:
1 tsp. cinnamon
1 to 2 packets Stevia, powdered
3 tbsp. water
1 medium apple

Directions:
Core and peel the apple and the dice it into half inch pieces.

Put the apple into a little crock pot or into a pot that has a lid.

Pour in the desired amount of cinnamon and the water.

Let the apples cook for around two hours set to low. The apples should be very soft. If you are cooking them on the stove, make sure you stir them every 20 to 30 minutes so that they don't stick to the pot.

Once the apples are done, mash them up with a fork or potato masher to your desired consistency.

Mix in the amount of Stevia that you want. Make sure you start with a little and taste along the way until it reaches your desired sweetness.

If you would like your applesauce to be really smooth, mix it up in a blender until it has become smooth. Enjoy.

Grilled Apple

Servings: 1
Phase 2

Ingredients:
1 tsp. of each:
lemon juice
Nutmeg
vanilla powder (this is optional)
1 to 2 packets Stevia
¼ tsp. cinnamon
1 apple

Directions:
Your oven should be at 375.

Remove the seeds and the core after slicing the apple in half.

Stir together the Stevia, vanilla powder (if using), nutmeg, and cinnamon. Make sure it is all mixed together well.

Sprinkle your apple halves with the spice mixture then put in the oven and cook for 13 to 15 minutes. The apples should be soft. The cooking time will vary depending on the size of your apple. Check the apples every five minutes so that they don't overcook. Top with lemon juice.

Heat up a grill and place the apples on a grill to get some nice char marks.

If you want a little more spice; add some extra cloves, nutmeg, or cinnamon. Enjoy.

Cinnamon Grapefruit

Servings: 1
Phase 2

Ingredients:
Water – if needed
1 to 2 packets Stevia, powdered
1 tsp. cinnamon
½ grapefruit

Directions:
Take a knife and your grapefruit and section the grapefruit. You want to take out as much of the pulp as you can. Run the knife around the inside of the grapefruit peel. Then run the knife between each grapefruit segment. After it has been loosened, turn the grapefruit upside down over a bowl and remove the segments. It's best just to get messy and pull the segments of pulp out.

Place all of the section in a small bowl. If you have a juicy grapefruit, then you won't have to mix in any water. If it seems to be dry, then sprinkle it with some water.

Sprinkle the grapefruit pieces with cinnamon and Stevia and toss it together.

Place the seasoned pieces back into the peel if you would like, and enjoy.

Apple Pie Crumble

Servings: 1
Phase 2

Ingredients:
1 medium apple
Crust:
2 tsp. water
¼ tsp. cinnamon
½ packet Stevia, powdered
½ grissini breadstick
Topping:
¼ tsp. cinnamon
½ packet Stevia, powdered
½ grissini breadstick

Directions:
Your oven should be at 350.

Core your apple and get rid of all the seeds. Chop the apple up into small pieces, around a quarter-inch. Place it to the side.

Put your breadstick in a bag and crush it up until it is in very small pieces.

Crust – Take the cinnamon, Stevia, and half of the breadstick crumbs and mix together. Slowly add some water until it starts to form a crumble topping.

Press your crust into the bottom of a small muffin tin or a soufflé dish.

Set the apple on top of your crust.

Topping – combine the topping ingredients together.

Place this mixture on top of your apple and bake it for around 15 to 20 minutes, or until the apple has softened up.

Take it out and enjoy.

Scotch Eggs

Servings: 6
Phase 4

Ingredients:

4 tbsp. oil
1 ½ c panko
1 beaten egg
¼ c flour
4 to 6 hard-boiled eggs, peeled and cooled
1 lb. breakfast sausage

Directions:

Your oven should be at 350. Split the sausage into four or six portions, depending on the number of eggs that you made and how thick you would like the sausage to be.

Flatten your sausage portions out and wrap them around each of your eggs to cover them.

Roll these balls in the flour, egg wash, and then into the panko.

Heat up some oil in a pan.

After it is hot, lower the heats and place in the eggs. Brown up the sides and place it on a rack that is set on a cookie sheet.

Set this in the oven for 20 to 40 minutes. Make sure that the sausage is cooked all the way through. If you choose to do all six eggs, you should only have to cook it for 20 minutes.

Enjoy immediately or keep it stored in the fridge.

Lunch

Shrimp and Wild Rice

Servings: 2
Phase 3

Ingredients:
½ tsp. of each:
onion powder
garlic powder
soy sauce
1 onion
2 tbsp. chicken stock
3 c water
1 tsp. salt
¼ c basmati rice, short-grain – if you have just entered phase 3 use orzo pasta
½ c wild rice – if you just entered phase 3 use orzo pasta
1 c shrimp

Directions:
It's recommended that you get medium-size pre-cooked shrimp from the frozen food area of your grocery store.
If you choose to use fresh shrimp, then boil it to cook it through before. Large shrimp will normally take around five to seven minutes while medium shrimp

will take around three to four minutes. If you have pre-cooked shrimp, allow them to completely thaw before using.

Slice the onion up into quarter-inch thick discs. Separate the onion sections.

Add the water, salt, and the rice or orzo into your pot. Let it come up to a boil. Stir, and then place a lid over it and let it simmer for around 40 to 45 minutes. The rice should be soft.

Set off the heat and get rid of any excess liquid.

Mix together the chicken stock and rice.

Stir in the soy sauce, garlic powder, onion powder, and shrimp.

Place a lid over and let everything warm up for around one to two minutes. Just make sure that the shrimp is warmed through.

Drain off excess liquid, and serve topped with onion.

Chicken Tacos

Servings: 1
Phase 2

Ingredients:

⅛ tsp. of each:
oregano
cumin
2 tbsp. cilantro, chopped
½ lemon
4 lettuce leaves
¼ tsp. cayenne
1 minced garlic clove
1 tsp. onion powder
100 grams chicken breast

Directions:

Remove off all of the visible fat from your chicken breast.

Set a pot of water on your stove and salt it. Allow the water to start boiling and add your chicken breast. Let the chicken cook until it reaches 165. Take the chicken out and let it cool off.

As your chicken cools off, get the lettuce ready. Make sure you wash and dry your lettuce before you use them to get rid of any pesticides that may be on them if you didn't buy organic.

Place the lettuce on a plate.

After the chicken has cooled off, shred the chicken up into smaller pieces with your hands.

Put the chicken into a pan and coat it with cumin, cayenne, oregano, garlic, and onion powder. Make sure it is mixed well.

Let the chicken heat back up for another three to five minutes. If the chicken sticks to the pan, add a little bit of water to it.

Set it off the heat and place your chicken over the lettuce. Top with some cilantro and squeeze of lemon juice. Enjoy.

Steak Spinach Salad

Servings: 1
Phase 4

Ingredients:

1 tbsp. powdered onion
2 minced garlic cloves
1 c tomato sauce – no sugar
2 tbsp. Italian seasoning
2 tsp. EVOO
1 flatbread wrap

Directions:

Your oven should be at 415.

Place the garlic, seasonings, and the tomato sauce into a small pot and mix it together.

Let the mixture heat up, making sure to stir it often.

While those cooks, take out your baking sheet or you could also use a pizza stone, then lay your flatbread on it.

Brush some olive oil on the flatbread then bake it for around three minutes. This will crisp it up so that it won't get so soggy.

Take the flatbread out and add on the tomato sauce. Make sure you spread it over it evenly.

Add your favorite cheese and the other toppings that you so desire.

Bake the pizza for another ten to 12 minutes. The cheese should be melted and starts to bubble. This will depend on what toppings you chose to use.

Take out of the oven and add a little extra Italian seasoning and cheese if you want. Enjoy.

Beef Patty Wrap

Servings: 1
Phase 2

Ingredients:

⅛ tsp. of each:
pepper
powdered garlic
powdered onion
salt
1 tbsp. sweet mustard dressing – HCG friendly
1 large lettuce leaf
100 grams ground beef, extra lean

Directions:

Since this is for phase two, make sure you have HCG approved ground beef. It should contain less than seven percent. Try to pick a meat that is 93/7 or 95/5.

Put your meat in a bowl and drizzle with the garlic powder, onion powder, pepper, and salt. Using your hands, mix all of the spices into the beef until mixed well.

Add the sweet mustard dressing and mix it through. Mold all of the meat mixtures into a patty. Compress it all together so that it will stay together while it cooks.

Place the patty into a pan. Once one side has browned up, flip it over and brown the other side. Add some water if the meat wants to stick to the pan. Continue to cook until it has cooked all the way through. Set it off the heat.

Place the lettuce leaf on a plate and set the patty on the leaf. Cover the patty with lettuce and enjoy with a little extra mustard dressing or regular yellow mustard.

Light Feta Salad

Servings: 1
Phase 3

Ingredients:
2 tbsp. low sugar and carb salad dressing
¼ c feta cheese, crumbled
4 to 5 baby carrots
¼ c cherry tomatoes
1 red bell pepper
½ cucumber
2 c spring lettuce mix

Directions:
Clean off all of the vegetables to remove any dirt or pesticides that may still be on them. This is very important to ensure what you eat it healthy.

Place the lettuce mix into a bowl.

You do not need to do this if you purchased crumbled feta. If you have a block, crumble it up with your hands and knife to make small crumbles.

Half the cucumber and dice into small pieces and add to your lettuce.

Make sure to wash and clean the pepper by removing its seeds and chop it up into small pieces and place it into your bowl.

Slice the tomatoes if you want and add to the salad.

Dice the carrots if you want to and add it to the salad.

Top your salad with your favorite dressing and toss everything together. Toss until everything has been completely coated.

Place on a plate and top with the cheese and pepper.

Tomato and Shrimp Kabob

Servings: 1
Phase 2

Ingredients:
Lemon Herb seasoning – Simple Girl
½ lemon, juiced
Pepper
Salt
¼ c tomatoes
100 grams shrimp

Directions:
If your shrimp are fresh, cook them thoroughly before you make your kabobs. Large shrimp will take around five to seven minutes, and medium shrimp will take around three to four minutes.

Cut the tomatoes in half. Cherry or grape tomatoes are the best to use because they hold their shape better when cooked. If you use a large tomato, then slice them into quarters.

Get your skewers ready. If you have wooden skewers, make sure that they have been soaked in water for around an hour, so that doesn't catch on fire.

Alternate the tomato and shrimp on your skewers.

If you want, sprinkle them with HCG safe seasoning. The Simple Girl is a good brand to go with.

Grill your skewer for two to three minutes on both sides. Make sure you don't end up smashing your tomatoes as you cook them. Since your shrimp should already be cooked, all you want to do is soften the tomatoes and give everything a grilled flavor.

Squeeze the fresh lemon juice over your skewer once done and enjoy.

Cod Salad

Servings: 1
Phase 2

Ingredients:
⅛ tsp. of each:
salt
pepper
1 grissini breadstick
2 tbsp. salad dressing – HCG friendly, optional
1 grissini breadstick
2 c baby spinach
1 tbsp. fresh lemon juice
¼ c chicken broth
100 grams white cod

Directions:
Your chicken broth should be homemade when in phase two of the HCG diet. You can also just use water if you don't have chicken broth.

Place the lemon juice and broth in a pot and heat.

Sprinkle pepper and salt over both sides of the cod.

When the broth mixture has heated, place the fish in and place on a lid. Allow the fish to cook until it is flaky and opaque.

Set it off the heat and let it cool slightly.

Clean your baby spinach to remove any pesticides, especially if not organic.

In a bowl, add the cod on top of the spinach. Pour the leftover broth mixture over your salad.

Serve this with a breadstick and enjoy.

Tomato and Steak Kabobs

Servings: 1
Phase 2

Ingredients:

1 tomato
1 tbsp. vinaigrette dressing
2 cloves garlic
½ tsp. salt
2 tbsp. oregano
100 grams sirloin steak, extra lean

Directions:

Slice the steak up into one-inch cubes.

Chop up the garlic finely, or press it through a garlic press.

Put the garlic, salt, oregano, dressing, and steak into a bag and shake it all together. Zip it closed and place it in the fridge for an hour.

Slice the tomato into quarters or cubes.

Get your skewers ready, soaking them if they are wood, so they don't catch on fire.

Place the meat and tomatoes on the skewers, alternating them.

Place them on your grill and let them cook for around two to three minutes on each side.

Set off the grill and enjoy.

Bison Patty

Servings: 1
Phase 2

Ingredients:
1 tbsp. sweet mustard dressing – HCG friendly
2 dill pickles
2 minced garlic cloves
1/8 tsp. onion powder
½ tsp. salt
2 tbsp. oregano
100 grams ground bison, lean

Directions:
Fold together the garlic, salt, onion powder, oregano, and bison. Using your hands form the meat mixture into one patty.

Heat up your grill. You can use an inside or an outside grill; anything works for this as long as you don't use oil.

Place the bison patty on your grill for around five to seven minutes on each side. The time may differ depending on how thick you made your patty.

Set the patty off to the side. Enjoy the patty with a couple of pickles spears and HCG friendly sweet mustard dressing.

Asian Cucumber salad

Servings: 1
Phase 2

Ingredients:
1 ½ tsp. red pepper flakes
¼ tsp. pepper
¼ tsp. salt
1 large cucumber
1 tsp. powdered garlic
8 drops Stevia
¼ c rice vinegar

Directions:
Clean your cucumber. This is extremely important especially if you do not buy organic produce. If, after washing it, the cucumber still looks waxy, you should probably peel it before you use it.

Chop up the cucumber into small pieces, small enough so that your food processor can hold it. Place everything from the list above into your food processor and pulse until the cucumbers have been chopped into tinier pieces.

This is faster with a food processor, but if you don't have one, then all you have to do is cut up the cucumber into tiny pieces and place in a bowl.

Put the spices, Stevia, and vinegar into a bowl and whisk them all together. Pour this mixture over your cucumber and enjoy.

BBQ Chicken Salad

Servings: 1
Phase 2

Ingredients:
1 grissini breadstick
2 tbsp. BBQ sauce – HCG friendly
2 c lettuce
1 tsp/ salt
100 grams chicken breast

Directions:
Trim off any extra fat that you can see on the chicken.
Put the chicken into a salted pot of water and let it boil until it is cooked all the way through.
Take the chicken out and let it cool.
Slice your lettuce into small pieces. This can be your favorite kind of lettuce. Romaine is a great option. Make sure you wash and dry your lettuce before you make your salad.
After the chicken has cooled, shred the chicken apart by hand.
Put the shredded chicken and the BBQ sauce into a bowl and toss together until the chicken is fully coated.
Place the lettuce into the chicken and toss everything together so that the lettuce gets covered in the sauce.
Serve your salad with a grissini breadstick.

Cucumber and Shrimp Salad

Servings: 1
Phase 2

Ingredients:
¼ tsp. of each:
red pepper flakes; crushed
salt
ground turmeric
½ tsp. pepper
½ lemon, juiced
2 minced garlic cloves
100 grams shrimp

Directions:
Wash off your cucumber before you chop it up. This is especially important if you didn't buy organic. If it still looks waxy after washing, you may want to peel it.

Combine the red pepper flakes, cumin, salt, pepper, garlic, and lemon juice together.

Put the lemon juice mixture and the shrimp in the same bowl and mix together. Place a lid on the bowl and let it chill for around an hour so that the spices mix together.

After its finished marinating, take it out of the fridge. Chop the cucumber up and then mix it into the shrimp.

Add some extra lemon juice if you want and enjoy.

Chicken Salad

Servings: 4
Phase 4

Ingredients:
2 tbsp. of each:
apple cider vinegar
Dijon mustard
½ tsp. of each:
celery seeds
pepper
1 tbsp. Stevia
3 tbsp. lemon juice
¼ tsp. salt
¼ c green onions, sliced
½ c sour cream
2/3 c mayonnaise
½ cup dried cranberries
2 cans water chestnuts
6 celery stalks
4 chicken breasts, cooked

Directions:
If you don't have any pre-cooked chicken, cook up some chicken in your favorite way, boiling is the quickest. Allow the chicken to cool before continuing.
Dice up the chicken breast.
Chop up the water chestnuts and celery.
Mix together the cranberries, water chestnuts, celery, and chicken in a big bowl and place to the side.
Mix the Dijon mustard, vinegar, sour cream, mayonnaise, and lemon juice in small bowl and add

the sweetener, pepper, and salt into the sauce and mix.

Stir in the green onions and celery seeds.

Top the chicken mixture with the dressing and toss everything together.

If you can wait, let it refrigerate for 30 minutes, so the flavors mix.

Cream of Chicken

Servings: 1
Phase 2

Ingredients:
¼ tsp. salt
¼ tsp. white pepper
½ tsp. basil
½ tsp. parsley
2 tsp. minced garlic
2 celery stalks
100 grams chicken breast
1 tbsp. milk
2 c chicken broth, or water

Directions:
Trim off all of the visible fat from the chicken and cook it in some salted water until done. Take out the chicken and allow it to cool. Once cooled, dice into cubes.

Put your water or chicken broth in a pot and let it start to heat up.

Chop up your celery.

Place the spices and milk into the broth then mix together. Stir it well so that all of the spices will be mixed together completely.

Add the chicken and celery.

Cover the pot then cook the chicken for 20 to 30 minutes. Stir it every once in a while.

Take it off from the heat and serve. Add extra pepper or salt if you need.

Chicken Wrap

Servings: 1
Phase 2

Ingredients:
2 to 3 lettuce leaves
1 tbsp. BBQ sauce, low carb
¼ tsp. salt
100 grams chicken breast

Directions:
Remove the visible fat from the chicken breast.

Place the chicken into a pot of water that has been salted and allow it to boil. Let the chicken cook until it is all the way done.

Set the chicken out and let it cool off so that you can handle it.

After the chicken has cooled, shred it up with your hands. Place it in a bowl and toss it with the BBQ sauce until it is completely coated.

Set you lettuce leaves out.

Lay the chicken on the lettuce and roll it together. Enjoy.

Grilled Shrimp Salad

Servings: 1
Phase 2

Ingredients:
⅛ tsp. of each:
salt
pepper
cumin
cayenne
1 grissini breadstick
2 tbsp. HCG safe dressing
2 c lettuce
100 grams medium shrimp

Directions:
Make sure you boil your shrimp if you choose to use fresh shrimp. Otherwise, purchase the frozen pre-cooked shrimp and make sure they are completely thawed.

If you are using wood skewers, make sure you soak them for around an hour. Place the shrimp on your skewers.

Mix the cayenne, cumin, pepper, and salt together. Sprinkle the mixture over your shrimp and rub it in.

Heat up whatever kind of grill that you want to use. Place the skewers on and sear both of the sides for a couple of minutes apiece. The shrimp is already cooked, so you are just doing this for the char and taste.

Set the shrimp over to the side.

Cut up your lettuce and place in a bowl. Top the lettuce with the shrimp and your HCG safe dressing. Toss all together and serve with the breadstick.

Dinner

Cauliflower Pizza

Servings: 1
Phase 3

Ingredients:
Basil leaves
2 tbsp. parmesan cheese, grated
¼ tsp. red pepper flakes; crushed
2 ½ c cauliflower, grated
1 ¼ c shredded mozzarella cheese
1 c grape tomatoes, sliced
¼ c tomato sauce
2 garlic cloves, sliced
Pepper
Salt
1 egg, beaten

Directions:
Your oven should be at 425. Place some parchment paper onto a baking sheet.

With a box grater, grate up the cauliflower until you have created two cups of cauliflower. Put the cauliflower into a bowl and let it microwave for seven to eight minutes. Once it's soft, take out so that it can cool.

Combine together the pepper, salt, parmesan, a cup of mozzarella, and egg and stir it into the cauliflower. Pat the mixture into a ten-inch circle onto your baking sheet. Spritz the top with cooking spray and put in the oven and cook for 10-15 minutes. It should turn golden on top.

Place the pizza sauce, the rest of the mozzarella, and the other toppings over the crust and bake for another ten minutes for the cheese to melt. Top with some basil if you would like.

Steak Spinach Salad

Servings: 1
Phase 2

Ingredients:
1 minced garlic clove
½ tsp. powdered onion
1 grissini breadstick
2 tbsp. salad dressing, topping – Simple Girl
2 c baby spinach
1 tbsp. salad dressing, marinade – Simple Girl
100 grams extra lean steak
⅛ tsp. of each:
sea salt
pepper

Directions:
Mince up your garlic until extra fine.

Put the steak into a baggie and add the tablespoon of salad dressing, onion powder, minced garlic, pepper, and salt. Zip it up and shake around to evenly coat. Place in the fridge for at least an hour. You can also prick the steak before marinating so that it can absorb the dressing easily.

Take the steak from the bag, and get rid of the leftover marinade.

Cook your steak either by baking or grilling, any method that keeps you from having to use cooking oil. Let it cook until it reaches your preferred doneness.

Clean your spinach and dry it. This is important to do so that it gets rid of all contaminants, especially if the spinach isn't organic.

After it dries, put it into a bowl with the steak and two tablespoons of your salad dressing.

Toss everything together and then pour out onto a plate.

Break up your grissini breadstick and place it on your salad. Enjoy.

Grilled Chicken and Corn

Servings: 1
Phase 3

Ingredients:
Salad:
1 c romaine, chopped
Your choice of vegetables
Corn:
1 to 2 tbsp. favorite dressing
Pepper
Salt
1 tbsp. melted butter
1 corn stalk
Chicken:
1 tsp. pepper
2 tbsp. EVOO
½ c all natural vinaigrette dressing
6 oz. chicken breast

Directions:
Marinate your corn and chicken in your favorite dressing. Let them sit for at least two hours.

Pierce your chicken with a fork several times to help it absorb the marinade easier.

Place all of the chicken ingredients together into a baggie and let marinate. Do the same with all of the corn ingredients.

While that marinates, mix together all of your salad dressing and place in the fridge for later.

Salt a pot of water and let it come up to a boil. Place the corn into the water and allow it to boil for eight to ten minutes. Set it off the heat once cooked, but leave it in the water while the chicken finishes cooking.

Heat up your grill until decently hot.

Take the chicken out of the bag and set it on the hottest part of the grill and let it cook for four minutes. If you want more char and grill marks, cook for two minutes with chicken sat at an angle on the grill. Rotate the chicken after two minutes and let it cook for two more. This will give your hash marks on your chicken.

Flip the chicken over and repeat the cooking until done.

Set it off the heat and let it cook for a couple of minutes so that all of the juices have time to redistribute.

While your grill is still hot, place the corn on the grill to give it some char marks. It won't take but a few minutes because the corn is already cooked.

Take it off the grill and brush with some melted butter and sprinkle with some pepper and salt.

Plate everything up with a side salad and add your favorite dressing to the salad.

Spaghetti

Servings: 1
Phase 3

Ingredients:
Parmesan cheese
2 basil leaves, garnish
Salt
Pepper
1 tsp. basil
1 tsp. Italian seasoning
2 tsp. oregano
1 garlic clove
½ small onion
16 oz. tomato sauce – sugar-free
1 lb. ground beef, lean
1 bag shirataki noodles

Directions:
Cook your noodles following the directions on the package.

Chop up your onion and breaking apart all of the layers.

If you want to, you can use store bought minced garlic once you are in phase three, but it's better to use regular garlic and mince it up on your own.

Place the beef in a skillet and brown it up. Make sure to break it apart as it cooks. Once it is cooked all the way through, place it into a pot and set it to the side.

In the same pan, place it back over the heat and add the onion and garlic. Cook them up until they have softened. Pour the onion and garlic into the pot with the beef.

Heat up the pot and add the pepper, salt, basil, Italian seasoning, oregano, and tomato sauce.

Place the lid over the pot and allow the mixture to cook for four to six minutes. Make sure you stir occasionally.

Take the pot off the heat and mix in the cooked noodles. Toss everything together.

Garnish with some basil and enjoy.

Vegetable Chili

Servings: 4
Phase 3

Ingredients:
½ c mushrooms
1 c chili beans, undrained
14.5 oz. tomato sauce, no-sugar added
14.5 oz. tomatoes, fire-roasted
1 tsp. pepper
1 tsp. salt
½ tsp. cumin
3 tbsp. red chili powder
1 tbsp. minced garlic
2 large carrots
1 bell pepper
½ onion
1 tbsp. EVOO
16 oz. ground beef, lean

Directions:
Chop up your peeled onion. Clean out the bell pepper and dice, matching the size of onion pieces. Mince up the garlic, and chop up the carrots.

Slice up your mushrooms and place them to the side. These will be added in at the very last of cooking.

Place your pot on the stove and add the spices, tomato sauce, tomatoes, and beans. Mix everything together and allow it to come up to a boil.

After it has begun to boil, place on its lid and let it simmer and cook for 35 to 45 minutes.

Place a pan on your stove and heat it up. Place in the garlic, carrots, bell pepper, onion, and ground beef. Let the mixture cook as you break up the beef until it is cooked all the way through.

Cook until the veggies have almost softened up.

In the last fifteen minutes of cooking add the beef, veggies, and mushrooms to your pot of chili. Mix them together and let them cook up until the mushrooms have become soft. Enjoy.

Mexican Steak

Servings: 1
Phase 3

Ingredients:
½ jalapeno
½ lime, juiced
1 handful cilantro
½ onion
1 tomato
¼ tsp. hot chili powder
1/8 tsp. salt
¼ tsp. pepper
1/8 tsp. garlic powder
1/8 tsp. cumin
6 oz. sirloin, lean

Directions:
To mix up your pico de gallo, mix together the jalapeno, lime juice, cilantro, onion, and tomato in your blender until it reaches your desired consistency. It should be runny though.

Stir together the chili powder, salt, pepper, garlic powder, and cumin and rub it over your steak. Let the steak sit for an hour or so if you can.

Heat up your grill until warm.

Place the steak on and sear both sides for around a minute.

Cover the steak and lower the temperature of the grill. Allow the steak to cook for another two to three minutes on each side. This will also depend on how done you want the steak and thickness of your piece of meat.

Set it off the heat and let it rest for a few minutes, so the juices redistribute.

Slice along the bias and top with your pico de gallo.

Seafood Gumbo

Servings: 1
Phase 2

Ingredients:
1/8 tsp. celery salt
1/8 tsp. garlic powder
¼ tsp. Creole seasoning
¼ tsp. onion powder
2 large tomatoes, chopped
1 chopped garlic clove
100 grams seafood – combination of white fish, lobster, scallops, or shrimp

Directions:
Cook up the seafood and mix in the garlic until it starts to brown up. Mix in all the other ingredients and let it simmer for about 15 minutes.

Blackened Salmon and Sweet Potatoes

Servings: 1
Phase 4

Ingredients:
Sweet Potatoes:
Pepper
Salt
1 tsp. milk
1 sweet potato
Salmon:
1 tbsp. butter – cooking
1 tbsp. butter – salmon
½ tsp. salt
½ tsp. pepper
¼ tbsp. garlic powder
¼ tbsp. cayenne
¼ tbsp. paprika
4 oz. salmon fillet

Directions:
Salmon – your oven should be at 350.
Mix all of the salmon spices together in a little bowl and place it to the side.
Melt a tablespoon of butter and brush the salmon with the butter.
Sprinkle the spices over the buttered salmon on all sides and put it in so that it sticks to the fish.
Heat a large pan and melt the remaining butter in the pan.

Set the salmon into the pan with skin side up. Let the bottom side sear for two to four minutes.

Places the salmon into a dish that is safe for the oven and let it bake for five to seven minutes, or until the salmon has cooked all the way through.

Sweet Potatoes – Cook you sweet potato either in the oven or the microwave until done. Allow it to cool.

Take the skin off of the potato and cut it into small pieces

Place the potato, pepper, salt, and milk into a bowl. Mash everything together with a fork or potato masher until it reaches your desired consistency.

Serve your salmon with the mashed sweet potato and a side salad topped with a low carb dressing.

Steak with Chili Sauce

Servings: 1
Phase 2

Ingredients:
8 oz. chili tomato sauce
¼ tsp. onion powder
1/8 tsp. cumin
3 minced garlic cloves
Steak seasoning – low carb and sugar
¼ tsp. pepper
1/8 tsp. salt
100 grams steak, extra lean

Directions:
Mince up your garlic cloves and place them to the side.

Heat up your grill to medium.

Place pepper and salt on your steak, and you can use a low carb steak seasoning if you wish to add more flavor. This way you will get the flavor of a steak house steak instead of a diet meal.

In a little pot, mix together the onion powder, cumin, garlic, and tomato sauce. Place a lid on the pot and let it cook softly for ten to 15 minutes. Stir often so that it doesn't burn.

Place your seasoned steak onto the hot grill and cook until the steak has cooked to your wanted level of doneness, and has browned on both sides.

Set the steak off the heat and let it cool off completely. After it is cooled, slice it into cubes.

Set the tomato off the heat and place in a bowl. Add the steak and more pepper and salt. Or you can dip the steak into the sauce.

Cinnamon Curry Chicken

Servings: 1
Phase 2

Ingredients:
1/8 tsp. pepper
1/8 tsp. salt
¼ tsp. pumpkin pie spice
¼ tsp. cinnamon
½ tsp. curry powder
3 minced garlic cloves
2 c chicken broth
1 medium onion
100 grams chicken breast

Directions:
The chicken broth that you use should be homemade.
Cook your chicken in some boiling water until it is completely cooked. You can also use leftover chicken if you have any. Trim all of the visible fat off.
Discard the water that the chicken was cooked in. Dice the chicken into cubes.
Place your pot back on the stove and add the chicken broth and all of the spices to your pot and mix well.
Dice up your onion and mix it into your pot.
Place the chicken into the pot and mix well. Place a lid on the pot and let it simmer and cook for 45 minutes.
Set it off the heat and let it cool for about five to ten minutes. Enjoy.

Turkey Meatball and Green Beans

Servings: 4
Phase 3

Ingredients:
2 c fresh green beans
¼ tsp. pepper
¼ tsp. salt
½ green bell pepper
2 garlic cloves
½ c parmesan cheese, grated
2 tbsp. parsley
1 onion, small
1 lb. ground turkey, extra lean

Directions:
Chop up your green bell pepper and onion.
Mince up the parsley and the garlic.
Place the pepper, salt, parmesan, and turkey meat into a bowl and mix it together with your hands. Add the chopped onion, pepper, garlic, and parsley. Combine together.
Form the meat into one-inch balls. Make sure they are rolled tightly so that they don't fall apart.
Set the meatballs on a wire rack set on a baking sheet. The baking sheet should be line with foil.
Your oven should be at 375.
Let the meatballs cook for 20 to 25 minutes. Cut one in half to make sure that they are done.
Allow them to cool for five minutes before serving.

Green beans – Cut the rough ends off and place them into a pan with a cup of water, just so that the beans are covered.

Place the lid on the pan and cook until the beans have become soft, or still have a little crunch, depending on how you like your green beans.

BBQ Chicken

Servings: 1
Phase 2

Ingredients:
Spinach
½ lemon, sliced
1/8 tsp. onion powder
1/8 tsp. garlic powder
1/8 tsp. pepper
1/8 tsp. salt
1 tbsp. BBQ seasoning, low carb
100 grams chicken breast

Directions:
You should place your oven on 350.

Cut all of the visible fat off of the chicken.

Season your chicken with the onion powder, garlic powder, pepper, and salt. Make sure you massage the spices into the chicken.

Put the chicken into a dish and cover with a lid. Place the chicken in the oven for 18 to 20 minutes.

Once 20 minutes have passed, take the lid off and bake for ten more minutes. The chicken should hit 165 degrees.

Immediately take the chicken out and coat with the BBQ seasoning.

Clean your spinach and place it on a plate. Top it with the chicken and a couple of wedges of lemon and enjoy.

Meaty Tomato Sauce

Servings: 1
Phase 2

Ingredients:
¼ tsp. pepper
¼ tsp. salt
¼ tsp. parsley
¼ tsp. oregano
¼ tsp. basil
¼ tsp. onion powder
¼ tsp. garlic powder
1 tsp. minced garlic
100 grams ground beef, extra lean
1 tbsp. water
1 large red tomato

Directions:
Dice up the tomato into small pieces.

Place the water and tomato into a pot. Place on the lid and let it cook for five to ten minutes. Stir it often so that it smashes up the tomato.

Let it cook until it has softened. Place tomato into a blender pulse everything up to your preferred consistency.

Place the mix back into the pot and mix in the pepper, salt, parsley, oregano, basil, onion powder, and garlic powder. Mix well and place on the lid. Let it cook for 20 to 30 minutes.

Cook the ground beef in a pan and break it apart as it cooks. Once it is cooked, mix it into the tomato sauce and let it cook for another five minutes.

Set it off the heat and enjoy.

Spinach Basil Pesto

Servings: 1
Phase 2

Ingredients:
HCG approved seasoning
100 grams chicken breast
1/8 pepper
1/8 tsp. salt
¼ tsp. oregano
1 lemon, juiced
1 tbsp. apple cider vinegar
3 garlic cloves
Handful basil
1 c baby spinach

Directions:
Mix the pepper, salt, oregano, lemon juice, and vinegar in a bowl and mix it together so that it combines.

Put the garlic cloves, basil, and spinach in a blender and pulse a couple of times until it is chopped up.

Slowly pour the lemon juice mixture into the blender as a steady stream while it's running.

Stop only to scrape the sides down so that everything gets mixed together well.

Pulse a couple more times to get everything together, and it is a paste-like consistency.

Pour the mixture into a serving bowl and place it to the side.

Remove all of the visible fat from your chicken. Season the chicken with HCG approved spices that you like.

Grill or bake you chicken once you have it seasoned. Make sure you can cook it without oil.

Once the chicken is cooked through, serve it on top of the pesto sauce. Enjoy.

Veal Parmesan

Servings: 1
Phase 2

Ingredients:
1 grissini breadstick
1/8 tsp. oregano
1/8 tsp. basil
1/8 tsp. pepper
1/8 tsp. salt
8 oz. Italiano sauce, HCG friendly

Directions:
Cut all of the visible fat from the veal.

Heat up your grill or pan.

Season your veal with some pepper and salt, rubbing it into the meat.

Once your grill or pan has heated up, place in the veal. Allow both sides to sear well. Turn the heat down and allow it to continue to cook until cooked to your liking.

While you veal is cooking, set a pot on the stove and mix in the oregano, basil, and Italiano sauce. If you choose to use fresh spices, make sure they have been minced up before you mix it in.

After the veal has cooked and your sauce is warm; pour the sauce on top of the veal.

Crush up the breadstick and sprinkle it over your veal. Enjoy.

Herbed Fish with Lettuce

Servings: 1
Phase 2

Ingredients:
3 to 4 lettuce leaves
1 grissini breadstick
1/8 tsp. pepper
1/8 tsp. salt
1 tbsp. oregano
2 tbsp. lemon juice, separated
100 grams white fish

Directions:
The lettuce you pick is up to you, but romaine works very well. Slice the lettuce into large chunks after you have washed and dried it.

Your oven should be at 400. Get a large piece of foil and lay it out and set the fish in the center. You can use any white fish that you like, which includes orange roughy, Whiting, tilapia, pock, burbot, sea bass, or cod.

In a bowl mix together the pepper, oregano, a tablespoon of lemon juice, salt.

Place the lemon mixture on top of your fish.

Fold up your foil and seal it up like a pouch.

Place the fish into your oven for ten to 20 minutes. The fish should flake.

Take it out and let it cool for a bit before you open it.

Lay the lettuce on a plate and set the fish on top. Add the remaining lemon juice on top.

Serve with the breadstick and enjoy.

Steak and Onion

Servings: 1
Phase 2

Ingredients:
Pepper
Salt
1 medium onion
1/8 tsp. red pepper flakes
1/8 tsp. cumin
1/8 tsp. chili powder
1 minced garlic clove
1/8 tsp. pepper
1/8 tsp. salt
100 grams steak, extra lean

Directions:
Slice the steak up into thin strips.

Set a skillet on top of your stove to get it warmed up for a few minutes.

Lay the steak into the hot skillet and immediately place in the pepper flakes, cumin, chili powder, garlic, pepper, and salt.

As the meat sears, chop your onions into small pieces.

After the steak has seared, mix in the onions and low the heat down. Allow this to cook, occasionally stirring, until the onions have become translucent. Let it cook until the meat has reached your preferred doneness.

Take it off the heat and place it on a serving dish.

Add some pepper and salt if you need to. Enjoy.

Sides

Tropical Fruit Salad

Servings: 4
Phase 3

Ingredients:
1 tbsp. orange juice, all natural
1 to 2 packets Stevia
1 small apple
¼ c watermelon
¼ c honeydew
¼ c pineapple
½ c grapes
1 kiwi fruit

Directions:
Peel your kiwi and then slice it into small slices and place into a bowl.

If you want, you can slice the grapes in half, and then place them into the bowl with the kiwi.

Core, peel, and chop up the pineapple into one-inch chunks and place into the bowl.

Peel and slice up the honeydew and watermelon and dice them into one-inch pieces, placing them into the bowl.

Core and peel the apple and dice into half inch pieces and add them into the bowl.

Sprinkle the Stevia over all the fruits and stir it all together.

Slowly add the orange juice and mixture well.

Place a lid onto the bowl and let it refrigerate for at least an hour so that everything combines and becomes juicy.

Enjoy.

Sweet and Spicy Cucumbers

Servings: 1
Phase 2

Ingredients:
1 tsp. sweet and hot seasoning
1 to 2 packets Stevia
1 cucumber

Directions:
Clean your cucumber up. This is important to remove all the pesticides from the skin. If it still looks waxy, peel your cucumber before you slice it up.

Slice your cucumber into 1/8 inch thick circles. Place the flat on a plate and add some sweet and hot seasoning onto the slices. If you don't want them too spicy, then limit how much of the seasoning you place on them.

Open you Stevia and sprinkle it over the cucumbers.

Place in the fridge to chill for ten to 15 minutes before you serve. The cucumbers are better when chilled.

Mixed Pepper Salad

Servings: 4
Phase 3

Ingredients:
½ tsp. garlic powder
½ tsp. onion powder
Pepper
Salt
1 tbsp. sesame oil
1 tbsp. apple cider vinegar
1 red bell pepper
1 orange bell pepper
1 yellow bell pepper
1 green bell pepper

Directions:
Deseed all of the peppers and dice them up into bite sized squares and place all of them into a bowl.

In a smaller bowl, mix together the garlic powder, onion powder, pepper, salt, sesame oil, and vinegar. Whisk it until it all comes together.

Pour this over you peppers and toss them together.

Place a lid on the bowl and place in the fridge to marinate for 45 to 60 minutes. This will help to soften up the peppers.

Stir again before serving.

Vitamin C Salad

Servings: 1
Phase 3

Ingredients:
1 tbsp. salad dressing
½ red bell pepper or orange
1 orange
½ c red grape tomatoes
1 carrot, peeled
1 c romaine lettuce

Directions:
Peel you orange and separate it into the segments.
Cut the rest of the ingredients into small bite sized pieces.
Put all of the ingredients into a bowl and top with your favorite low carb and sugar salad dressing.
Toss all of the ingredients together and enjoy.

Basil Vinaigrette

Servings: varies
Phase 2

Ingredients:
1 garlic clove
Handful basil
½ packet Stevia
½ tsp. onion powder
½ tsp. pepper
½ tsp. salt
¾ c cold water
1/3 c apple cider vinegar

Directions:
Chop up the basil and garlic roughly.
Place the basil and garlic into your blender. Place all the other above ingredients into your blender and mix it together until it becomes a liquid consistency. If your dressing looks thick, add a little bit of water.

Citrus Vinaigrette

Servings: varies
Phase 2

Ingredients:
Dash pepper
1/8 tsp. salt
1 garlic clove
¼ tsp. onion powder
1 tbsp. lemon juice
2 tbsp. apple cider vinegar
1 tbsp. orange juice, fresh

Directions:
Slice your orange in half and juice it to get the juice you need for the dressing.

Mix together the lemon juice, vinegar, and orange juice.

Mix in the pepper, salt, garlic, and onion powder into the liquid ingredients.

Mix everything together well. It's best that you keep it in a shaker jar because you will need to shake it before using it.

Apple Cider Dressing

Servings: varies
Phase 2

Ingredients:
1/8 tsp. pepper
1/8 tsp. sea salt
1 to 2 packets Stevia, powdered
1/3 c apple cider vinegar
2/3 c water

Directions:
Whisk together the vinegar and water until well combined.
Mix in the Stevia until it has completely dissolved.
Whisk in the pepper and salt and pour it into a shaker jar. It will need to be shaken before you use it.

Chicken Celery Soup

Servings: 1
Phase 2

Ingredients:
1 grissini breadstick
¼ tsp. pepper
¼ tsp. salt
¼ tsp. cayenne
1 bay leaf
½ tsp. poultry spice
2 c celery
2 minced garlic cloves
100 grams chicken breast
2 c chicken broth – or water

Directions:
Put your water or chicken broth in a pot and let it begin to heat up.

Mix in the pepper, salt, cayenne, bay leaf, and poultry spice into the water, and let this come up to a boil.

While the broth is heating up, trim off all the fat that you can see from the chicken breast.

Once the broth has started to boil, add the chicken breast. Allow this to cook until the chicken breast has cooked all the way through. Take the chicken out and let it cool off.

Once you can handle it, shred it up or dice it into small pieces.

Mince your garlic and dice of the celery. Place the chicken, garlic, and celery into the pot and stir to distribute.

79

Place the lid on the pot and turn the temperature to a simmer. Allow this to cook for another 20 minutes. The celery should be tender.

Set it off the heat and fish out the bay leaf. Add more pepper and salt if you need to.

Enjoy with your breadstick.

Creamy Pasta

Servings: 2
Phase 3

Ingredients:
Water
1/8 tsp. salt
1/8 tsp. pepper
1 tsp. onion powder
1 tsp. garlic powder
1 c broccoli
1/8 c pesto sauce
¼ c parmesan cheese
1 c Greek yogurt, unsweetened and plain
1 bag shirataki noodles

Directions:
Follow the directions on your noodle package, and fully cook them. Place them to the side.

Chop up your broccoli and place them in a large pot.

Add enough water to the bottom of the pot so that its bottom is covered completely.

Place a lid on the pot and allow the broccoli to steam for three to six minutes.

After the broccoli has reached your desired softness and set it off the heat. Drain all of the water out of the broccoli and allow it to cool.

Place all of the seasonings, pesto sauce, parmesan, and yogurt to the pot.

Place the mixture on your lowest heat setting and let it cook for two to three minutes. You should make sure to stir often. Don't let the mixture overheat.

If your sauce becomes too thick, add some water, a teaspoon at a time, until it reaches a good consistency. Stir in the noodles and the broccoli and mix until everything is coated.

Set it off the heat and place it in a serving dish.

Top with some extra cheese and pepper if you want.

Chinese Stir-Fry

Servings: 1

Phase 3

Ingredients:

1 tbsp, soy sauce

1 tbsp, rice vinegar

Packet Stevia, powdered

1 tbsp, peanut butter

1 carrot, sliced

½ c mushrooms, sliced

½ c green bell peppers, sliced

1 c broccoli, chopped

7 oz bag shirataki noodles

Directions:

Cook your noodles according to the directions on the bag.

Combine the soy sauce, vinegar, Stevia, and peanut butter together in a little bowl.

Pour the sauce into a pan and let it cook for about a minute or two.

Mix in the carrots, bell peppers, and broccoli, tossing to coat the veggies. Let the mixture cook for five to seven minutes.

Make sure you stir the mixture often so that it doesn't stick.

Mix in the mushrooms and cook until they have softened up.

Toss the cooked noodles with the sauce mixture and coat. Enjoy.

Artichoke Salad

Servings: 1
Phase 3

Ingredients:
2 tbsp. salad dressing – low carb and sugar
1 tsp. capers – optional
4 to 5 c yellow tomatoes
¼ c red tomatoes
½ c artichoke hearts – non-marinated
1 c romaine lettuce
1 c red leaf lettuce

Directions:
Slice all the lettuce up into bite sized pieces. Chop up all of the tomatoes. Place the tomatoes and lettuce into a bowl.

If the artichoke heart you bought isn't already quartered, slice them into quarters.

Place the hearts and capers into the bowl with the lettuce and tomatoes.

Top with your favorite low carb salad dressing. Toss everything together and enjoy.

Dill Cucumber Salad

Servings: 1
Phase 2

Ingredients:
¼ tsp. salt
¼ tsp. pepper
1 to 2 packets Stevia
1 tsp. Dill seasoning
1 tsp. apple cider vinegar
1 large cucumber, you should have a two cups

Directions:
Begin by washing your cucumber, making sure to clean it well. If it still appears waxy, you may want to peel it first.

Slice the cucumbers into quarters and then chop the quarters into chunks and set to the side.

Place the pepper, salt, Stevia, Dill, and apple cider vinegar in a bowl and mix together.

Make sure you stir until the Stevia has completely dissolved.

Toss the cucumbers in the mixture. Season with extra pepper and salt if you need to and enjoy.

Chicken Broth

Servings: varies
Phase 2

Ingredients:
½ tsp. salt
¼ tsp. pepper
¼ tsp. poultry seasoning
¼ tsp. celery salt
¼ tsp onion powder
¼ tsp. garlic powder
8 c water
6 pieces of chicken breast

Directions:
Place the pepper, salt, poultry seasoning, celery salt, onion powder, garlic powder, and the water to a big pot.

Mix everything together so that the spices dissolve.

Place the chicken into the pot and allow the mixture to come up to a boil.

Once it has started boiling, place the lid on the pot and turn down the heat.

Let it cook until the chicken is cooked through.

Take out the chicken and reserve for some other use.

Store the broth in a jar to use with many of the recipes in this cookbook.

Appetizers and Desserts

Apple Topia

Servings: 1
Phase 3

Ingredients:
1 packet Stevia
1 tsp. cocoa powder, unsweetened
2 tbsp. peanut butter
1 apple

Directions:
Slice up your apple into quarter-inch thick disks.

Cut out the core from the center of each of the apple disks. Place these disks to the side.

Mix together the Stevia, cocoa, and peanut butter until it comes together.

If your peanut butter is thick and stirring is hard, add a bit of water to the mixture to help soften things up.

Taste the mixture to see if you need to add some more Stevia.

Set the bottom apple piece onto a plate and smear it with the peanut butter mixture. Place the next disk on top and continue to layer the peanut butter and apple pieces. Enjoy.

Peppermint Mocha

Servings: 1
Phase 2

Ingredients:
7 drops chocolate Stevia
7 drops peppermint mocha Stevia
1 c hot water

Directions:
Heat up your cup of water, either on the stove or in the microwave. Mix in all of the Stevia and enjoy.

Miracle Noodle Cookie

Servings: varies
Phase 3

Ingredients:
1/8 tsp. sea salt
2 packets Stevia, powdered
½ tsp. vanilla
½ tsp. baking powder
3 tbsp. cocoa powder, unsweetened
2 eggs
8 to 9 oz. bag shirataki noodles

Directions:
Follow the directions for your pack of shirataki noodles.

After you have cooked your noodles, dry them completely. If they aren't completely dried, then you run the risk of having runny cookie dough.

Set the noodles in the fridge to cool for ten to 15 minutes.

After the noodles are cool and dry, put them into your blender and pulse them for 30 to 45 seconds.

Add the cocoa powder and eggs, and pulse them together until they are combined.

Add the salt, Stevia, vanilla, baking powder to the blender and mix them all together.

Remove the dough from the blender and form them into half an inch sized cookie balls.

Place some parchment paper on a cookie sheet and set the cookie dough balls onto the cookie sheet.

Your oven should be at 375.

Place the cookies into the oven and check to see if they are done at eight minutes. Don't cook any longer than ten minutes.

When the edges have firmed up, take them out of the oven.

Let them cool and then enjoy.

Tomato Mint Salsa

Servings: 1
Phase 2

Ingredients:
Pepper – to taste
Salt – taste
1 tsp. onion powder
½ tsp. garlic powder
1 lemon, juiced
1 bunch mint, minced
1 minced garlic clove
1 large tomato

Directions:
Chunky – Mince up the tomato, garlic clove, and mint leaves. Put all of your chopped ingredients into a bowl, with the juice from the tomato. Top everything with some fresh lemon juice. Mix in the pepper, onion powder, salt, and garlic powder. Stir everything together and enjoy.

Smooth – Place all of the ingredients from above, including the spices, into your food processor or blender. Pulse everything together until it reaches your desired consistency.

Creamy Coffee

Servings: 1
Phase 2

Ingredients:
5 to 6 ice cubes
6 drops chocolate Stevia
6 drops vanilla Stevia
1 tbsp. milk, your favorite
1 c brewed black coffee

Directions:
Allow your coffee to cool off and mix in the Stevia drops and milk. Make sure you stir it well so that the Stevia flavors are well mixed.

Pour over some ice if you would like, and enjoy.

Steak Spinach Salad

Servings: 1
Phase 2

Ingredients:
5 drops chocolate Stevia
5 drop English toffee Stevia
1 c coffee
1 c ice

Directions:
Brew yourself a plain cup of coffee.

Once the coffee has brewed, allow it to cool off completely. Don't use ice to make it cool off faster because this will only make the coffee watered down. This will ruin the flavor of the coffee.

After the coffee is cold, mix in the Stevia, and ice and stir together.

If you want, you can pour it into a blender and combine together. Enjoy.

Hot Apple Cider

Servings: 1
Phase 2

Ingredients:
Water – as needed
1 to 2 packets Stevia
Dash ground cloves
Dash nutmeg
Dash allspice
¼ tsp. cinnamon
½ tbsp. apple cider vinegar
2 tbsp. lemon
1 medium apple, freshly juiced

Directions:
Put the fresh apple juice in a pot with the lemon juice, and apple cider vinegar, and mix well.

Stir in the Stevia, cloves, nutmeg, allspice, and cinnamon. Whisk to help get everything incorporated. Place a lid on the pot and let it cook for a bit on low.

Give a bit of taste test to see if you need to add water to dilute the flavors. Go by your taste in deciding the strength of your cider.

Place in a mug once warm and enjoy.

Lemonade

Servings: 1
Phase 2

Ingredients:
Ice
2 to 3 packets Stevia, powdered
1 lemon, juiced
16 oz. water

Directions:
Remove the seeds from the freshly squeezed lemon juice if there is any and place into a large glass.

Stir in the Stevia until it is completely dissolved. It is always best to start with less Stevia and taste it to see if you need to add more. You don't want it to be too sweet.

Mix in the water, and make sure everything is well incorporated.

Pour the lemonade over ice and enjoy.

Classic Cucumber Salad

Servings: 1
Phase 2

Ingredients:
½ tsp. pepper
½ tsp. salt
3 to 4 ice cubes
2 tbsp. apple cider vinegar
1 large cucumber

Directions:
Wash up your cucumber. If it still appears shiny or waxy after it has been washed, you may want to peel it to remove any harmful chemicals.

Slice up the cucumbers into 8-inch thick discs and place them into a bowl.

Pour the apple cider vinegar into the cucumbers so that they are covered.

Mix in the pepper, salt, and ice cubes.

Set it in the fridge and allow it to chill for around ten minutes. These taste better when they are extremely cold.

Take them out and remove any of the ice cubes.

Add more pepper and salt if you need to and enjoy.

Homemade Salsa

Servings: 1
Phase 2

Ingredients:

Cayenne pepper, to taste – optional
½ packet Stevia, powdered – optional
½ tsp. pepper
½ tsp. salt
1 tbsp. cilantro
1 tsp. onion powder
¼ tsp. oregano
2 minced garlic cloves
1 tbsp. lemon juice
1 medium tomato

Directions:

Chop up the tomato into small pieces; you can remove the core and seeds if you want. Add your lemon juice and toss together.

Mince up the garlic and place them with the tomato.

Take your cilantro and finely chop it up, making sure you don't use the stem. Mix it into the tomato.

Place in the pepper, salt, onion powder, and oregano and toss it all together.

Now is the time to give it a taste to see if you need to adjust any flavors. If you want your salsa a little sweet, and some Stevia. You can also add some cayenne if you want it a bit spicier.

Stir everything together and enjoy.

Conclusion

Thanks for making it through to the end of *The HCG Diet Cookbook*. Let's hope it was informative and able to provide you with all of the tools you need to achieve your goals.

The next step is to make the commitment to change your body and life for the better. Get started on your diet and use the recipes in this book to help you through this diet.

Finally, if you found this book useful in any way, a review on Amazon is always appreciated!

HCG Diet

The Step by Step Guide to Rapid Fat Loss,
Laser Sharp Focus, and a Better Life

Michelle Jones

The following eBook is reproduced below with the goal of providing information that is as accurate and as reliable as possible. Regardless, purchasing this eBook can be seen as consent to the fact that both the publisher and the author of this book are in no way experts on the topics discussed within, and that any recommendations or suggestions made herein are for entertainment purposes only. Professionals should be consulted as needed before undertaking any of the action endorsed herein.

This declaration is deemed fair and valid by both the American Bar Association and the Committee of Publishers Association and is legally binding throughout the United States.

Furthermore, the transmission, duplication or reproduction of any of the following work, including precise information, will be considered an illegal act, irrespective whether it is done electronically or in print. The legality extends to creating a secondary or tertiary copy of the work or a recorded copy and is only allowed with express written consent of the Publisher. All additional rights are reserved.

The information in the following pages is broadly considered to be a truthful and accurate account of facts, and as such any inattention, use or misuse of the information in question by the reader will render any resulting actions solely under their purview. There are no scenarios in which the publisher or the original author of this work can be in any fashion deemed liable for any hardship or damages that may befall them after undertaking information described herein.

Additionally, the information found on the following pages is intended for informational purposes only and should thus be considered, universal. As befitting its nature, the information presented is without assurance regarding its continued validity or interim quality. Trademarks that are mentioned are done without written consent and can in no way be considered an endorsement from the trademark holder.

Table of Contents

Introduction

Congratulations on downloading this book and thank you for doing so.

The following chapters will discuss some of the basics of the hCG (Human Chorionic Gonadotropin) diet. This diet plan is a fantastic way to lose weight quickly without a ton of effort. Simply taking an injection of the hCG hormone and cutting down your calories (which you will be able to do on this diet without losing energy or starving), you can lose up to two pounds each day that you maintain this diet plan.

This guidebook is going to provide you with all the information that you need in order to get started on the hCG diet. We will talk about what the hCG diet is along with some of the health benefits from this diet plan. The hCG diet is then split up into three phases and each one is important in helping you lose a lot of weight. So, we will take some time to discuss each of the phases so that you are able to complete them successfully. The final chapters will talk about the importance of working out on this diet plan and even how to maintain the results when you are all done.

There are quite a few diet plans on the market that you can choose from and some of them can give you amazing results. But none will work as well as the hCG diet. Take some time to read through this guidebook and learn everything that you need to know to get started.

There are plenty of books on this subject on the market, thanks again for choosing this one! Every effort was made to ensure it is full of as much useful information as possible, please enjoy!

Chapter 1: What is the HCG Diet?

There are many different types of diet plans that you can pick. Some will ask you to fast part of the time in the hopes of increasing your fat burning hormone. Some ask you to cut out all the fats and just focus on the carbs and healthy produce while others will go the other way and cut out all the carbs while eating healthy fats. And there are so many different diet plans in between.

The hCG (Human Chorionic Gonadotropin) diet is a bit different compared to the other ones. The idea behind this diet plan is to take a hormone that is naturally produced in the body during pregnancy, to help you lose weight. The promise of this diet plan is that when you increase your levels of this hormone, you will be able to lose weight quickly. In addition, if you add these natural hormones with a diet that is really low in calories, you will be able to reset the metabolism while losing a pound or more each day, without all the hunger and deprivation.

So, does this diet plan work? According to science, any diet that restricts your calories to super low levels will end up resulting in weight loss. Adding in the hCG hormone may help to increase the weight loss more than just eating a low-calorie diet is able to do.

You will find that this diet will really limit how many calories that you are able to consume on a regular day, much more than you are used to consuming. For example, for the eight weeks that you are taking the hormone, you will need to keep your calorie count around 500 for the whole day. In addition to keeping the calories low, you will take in the hormone through a shot or some other homeopathic product like sprays, pellets, or oral drops.

It is important to remember that while you may be able to lose a lot of weight on this diet plan, none of the homeopathic methods of getting the hCG are approved for weight loss by the FDA. The shots are legal, but you do need to make sure that a health care provider gives them to you and usually they are used to help out with fertility issues. But any product that is sold over the counter for hCG is not considered legal so be careful and do your research before picking out the product that you will use.

The main part that you will need to concentrate on when choosing this diet plan is to take in the hCG hormone each day for the eight weeks and to make sure that your calorie count stays low. If you are able to keep these two things in line, you will be able to lose up to a pound each day on the diet.

The food basics of this diet plan

While there are some specific rules about what you are able to eat on the hCG diet, basically you will not eat too much on this plan. The diet will let you eat for two meals each day, during lunch and during dinner, but your meals need to be small so that they fit inside the 500-calorie limit. Each meal that you eat needs to have one fruit, one bread, one vegetable, and one protein.

There are some restrictions on the way that you are able to eat the foods that you want to have. For example, as long as you are able to get rid of the fat that is visible on the meat, you are able to grill or boil shrimp, crab, lobster, white fish, chicken breast, beef, veal. Keep the portions low on these so that you can keep your calorie count and get in the two meals.

Since vegetables are pretty low in calories, you can have a few more of these and still stay on the diet plan. Some of the choices that you can make with vegetables and still be on the hCG diet include cabbage, asparagus, cucumbers, red radishes, onions, fennel, celery, tomatoes, green salad, beet greens, and spinach.

For bread, you are going to be pretty limited on the choices that you have. Most grain choices are going to be higher in calories so you have to be careful not to let them eat up all the calories that you are allowed to have. Your bread allowance for the meals will include a small piece of Melba toast or a small breadstick.

Your choices with fruits are going to be a little bit more limited as well. There are a lot of fruits that are high in calories and sugars so you need to keep them down to a minimum. You are able to have half a grapefruit, a small handful of strawberries, an apple or an orange for one of your servings with each meal.

There are a few other things that you are able to consume when you are on the hCG diet. You are able to choose as much tea, coffee, and water as you would like. You can add a bit of milk to your coffee, but you can only have a tablespoon of the milk every day so don't add in a ton. Sugar substitutes are fine on this diet plan, but never use sugar as a way to sweeten your drinks. Oils and butter will not be allowed on this diet plan.

Taking the hCG

In addition to focusing on the food that you are allowed to eat on the hCG diet, and remember that you need to keep the calorie count at 500 or below for the whole 8 weeks, you also have to take in the hCG hormone to see the results that you would like.

There are a few methods that you are able to use to take the hCG hormone. If your doctor has recommended that you go on a low-calorie diet to help with your high blood pressure or to help you fight obesity, you will be able to get the shot from them. This is often the safest method of getting the hormone since you are getting it from a trained professional.

There are some people who would like to go on this diet but who may not meet the conditions that are needed to get approval from your doctor. There are a few other methods that you can use. You can choose to take a pill or a spray. There are some homeopathic options that you can use. You will need to make sure that you take them at the right times and right amounts during the three phases of the hCG diet so that you can get the best results.

Is the hCG diet hard?

Compared to a lot of the other diet plans that are available for you to choose from, the hCG diet is really hard to stick with. Not only do you need to remember to take in the hCG hormone each day, but the calories are really restricted. It can be really hard to only eat 500 calories each day and depending on how good you are at planning your meals out, you could miss out on some of your nutritional needs as well.

Most doctors and nutritionists agree that it is almost impossible to get enough protein, fat, carbs, and other minerals and vitamins in each day without consuming at least 1200 calories each day. This is what our bodies need just to function and going too far below that will make it hard to function for too long. Some people who go on this diet take in supplements to help them meet this nutritional void.

If you do decide to go on this diet plan, you need to be aware of the nutritional needs that your body requests. It is not good enough to eat a few donuts and call that your 500 calories for the day. This will harm the body and make it almost impossible to stick with the diet. This diet is hard enough, don't make it worse by not providing the body with the nutrition that it needs.

Since this diet is so restrictive and hard for some people to follow, it is usually only recommended for those who really need to lose a lot of weight in order to regain their health. If you are severely obese and are facing issues like heart failure, diabetes, high blood pressure, and other conditions and you need to react quickly, the hCG diet can be the right one for you. You do need to be prepared and understand that this diet plan is going to take some hard work and dedication on your part.

There are a few times when a doctor will recommend a diet that is very low in calories. This means that the diet will be under 1000 calories, similar to what is required with the hCG diet. If someone is obese or they are dealing with a health condition that could be improved with losing weight, they may recommend a diet like this for their patients. But all of these diets need to be supervised. Make sure that when you pick out a diet like the hCG diet, you really need it, not that you choose it to just lose a few vanity pounds.

What if I cheat on the hCG diet?

The hCG diet can be a really hard one for you to follow. You need to cut down on the amount of calories that you consume down to just 500. The hCG hormone will help out with this one so that you won't always feel hungry, but trying to figure out which meals you will eat on this small calorie limit can be impossible some days. Add in that you need to make sure that the meals not only fit in with your calorie allowance but that they provide you with the nutrition you are looking for.

Because the diet can be really hard to follow, you need to be aware that you may be tempted to cheat. If you cheat on one of your meals, it is time to reorganize, but it is not the end of the world. Do not go into it thinking that since you already cheated you are able to cheat for the rest of the day. Recognize that the cheat happened and learn from the mistake, but try to organize the rest of the day so that you still end up within the guidelines of the hCG diet.

Often the biggest reason that people will cheat on the hCG diet is that they did not plan enough ahead of time. Before you go on this diet, consider getting a few different recipes in line and have the ingredients on hand. Then you know that all of the ingredients around you are just fine. Even making some of the meals ahead of time so that you can just throw them in when it is time to eat can take away some of the struggles when dinner time comes around. When a lot of the work is done ahead of time, it takes away the stress, and the temptation, that can come when it is time to make meals.

Exercising on the hCG Diet

Exercising is very important when it comes to the hCG diet. This is going to help you to see even more weight loss than before and will set you up for a healthier lifestyle once you are done with the three phases of the hCG diet. It is important that you pick out the right types of exercise though.

Doing exercises that are high intensity will not be good on this particular diet plan. When this is combined with the low calories you will consume, the body will presume that you are under stress and will start to store fat. This kind of defeats the purpose of going on the hCG diet to lose weight and to burn off fat. Pick out lower intensity workouts like swimming, light strength training, brisk walking, and yoga instead. You can add in the higher intensity options once you are done with the diet plan if you want.

The hCG diet can be a very effective method of losing weight quickly. It has claims that you can lose up to a pound each day that you are on the diet plan, which lasts for eight weeks, as long as you restrict your calories and take in the hCG hormone each day. This could be the answer you are looking for when you need to improve your health and lose weight quickly.

Chapter 2: What are the Benefits of the HCG Diet?

When you get started on a new diet plan, you want to make sure that you pick one that can provide you with the best benefits possible. There are so many options that are available, you want to make sure that you pick out one that is truly effective at helping you to lose weight and provide you with some other health benefits. And with how difficult the hCG diet can be over the eight weeks, you really want to make sure that you gain as many benefits as possible. This chapter will take some time to look over the benefits of the hCG diet and why you should choose this diet plan for your weight loss goals.

There are many benefits that come with going on the hCG diet. The first one is that this diet plan will help you to reach full energy levels. Even though you will reduce your calorie intake over these eight weeks, you will find that the hCG hormone is able to increase your energy levels. Nothing is better than being able to lose your weight while also having lots of energy in the process.

While it may seem a bit hard to go on the hCG diet and restrict your calorie count down to 500 or less each day, you will not feel tired or hungry. There are some other diet plans that will restrict your calories quite a bit, but they don't have the secret weapon that helps you to feel full and satisfied, even with a lower calorie intake.

Another concern that some people will have when they restrict their calorie intake for a longer period of time (longer than a day or two when they are sick), is that this will cause issues with blood sugar levels. The hCG hormone will help you out with this, keeping your blood sugar levels safe and stable throughout the whole time. This is actually a good diet to go on if you are trying to fight off diabetes because it does help to stabilize your blood sugars.

Since you are taking the hCG hormone, which is going to help speed up your metabolism, and you are reducing your calorie intake, you will be able to lose weight. But what is even better is that your weight loss is going to happen in the tough areas of the body, the areas where fat will store and is hard to burn off. The hCG diet is one of the most effective diets that you are able to pick that helps with burning off the fat.

The hCG diet can be nice because it will help to preserve your muscle integrity. Many times, when you go on a low-calorie diet similar to this one, you have to worry about the muscles not getting enough nutrients. Sometimes, there will be weight loss, but the weight loss is not from fat, but from muscle. The hCG hormone is able to help preserve the muscles so that you actually lose weight that matters.

One of the claims that comes with the hCG diet is that it can help to improve the functioning of your metabolism. Over the years, the American diet can do a number on how well the metabolism is going to work. It is likely your metabolism is running slowly and this can make losing weight almost impossible. With the help of the hCG hormone and following the right diet plan, you can get your metabolism up and working again.

For men, there is the added benefit of having a higher level of testosterone while on this diet plan. This can be great for those who would like to gain muscle mass while working out on this diet plan. For women, they will get the added benefit of estrogen levels that are more controlled. This is part of the reason that the hCG hormone shot is offered for those who are suffering from fertility issues. The hCG hormone can help to keep the estrogen levels more controlled so it is easier to have regular cycles and become pregnant.

No matter what group you are in, you will find that the hCG diet can help you to develop some healthier eating habits. You will not go on this diet for the rest of your life, which means that you will be able to increase your calorie intake at some point. But while you are on the hCG diet, your calories need to come from good and healthy foods so that you can provide the body with healthy nutrients while on a limited calorie diet.

While the typical American diet is high in fats, sugar,

and processed foods, along with other ingredients that can harm the body, the hCG diet will allow you to eat healthier and more wholesome foods. You can then take some of these new eating habits that you learned and translate them over when you increase your calorie goals after the diet.

But one of the biggest benefits that you will see when you choose to go on the hCG diet is the huge amounts of weight loss. There are a lot of diet plans that promise some good weight loss benefits, but none are as effective over a short amount of time as the hCG diet. In fact, if you take the hormone and stick with the calorie restrictions correctly, it is possible to lose a pound each day while on this diet plan.

This kind of weight loss is hard to maintain over the long term, but since the hCG diet is just for eight weeks, it is something that you will be able to enjoy. This is why those who are severely obese or who need to lose weight quickly to help out with their health conditions will choose to go on the hCG diet. This diet plan helps them to lose weight quickly and efficiently, without feeling hungry or deprived, so they can gain back their own good health.

There are so many great benefits that come with the hCG diet and it is hard to just pick one reason why you would want to start. Take a look through some of the phases that you will need to follow to be successful on the hCG diet, and you will be ready to lose weight.

Chapter 3: Phase One of the HCG Diet

When you get started on the hCG diet, there are going to be three main phases that you can follow. Following these phases will make it easier for you to get the results that you want and will make sure that you are burning off as much of that unwanted fat as you can. First, we will start with some of the things that you should have in order before you get started on this diet plan and then move on to some of the basics of the first phase of the hCG diet.

Getting Started

Being prepared is one of the best things that you can do to get started on the hCG diet plan. You want to make sure that you have everything in order so that you can make the best decisions possible. Some of the things that you may want to consider purchasing ahead of time so they are on hand include:

A good scale: you don't have to purchase the most expensive scale that you can find, but make sure it is not a used one at a garage sale either. Every morning during the diet you will need to weigh yourself so that you can record your progress. If your scale is not accurate, it is going to be hard to catch some of the fluctuations that may happen in your diet, and you won't be able to make the right corrections.

Food scale: you will need to carefully measure out the food portions that you eat. This will ensure that you keep your calorie goals where they should be during this diet plan. You will need to measure your vegetables, fish, meats, and more. You should always weigh your ingredients raw before you prepare the meals.

hCG: it is hard to follow the hCG diet if you are not going to take the hCG hormone. Make sure to find the version of this hormone that will work the best for you and consider getting enough to keep on hand for the full time of the diet.

Ketone sticks: these are not necessary on the diet, but can be a welcome addition. You will be able to find them at a lot of the health and drug stores in your area. These will be good to check out how well the body is processing fat during the diet. Again, you can choose whether you would like to have these around or not.

Grill: all of the protein that you consume on this diet plan needs to be broiled, grilled, or steamed, so if you don't already have a grill handy, you may want to consider finding one. George Foreman grills can be a nice option or you can pick the one that you would like.

Before you get started on the hCG diet, you need to make sure that you are comfortable with portion control during meals. You are only allowed to have 500 calories and this does need to be split up between two different meals during the day, so understanding how big your portions can be before starting will make a big difference. While eating food is going to be different in terms of calories, make sure to understand how much is in each one and use your scale so that you stay within your limits.

Phase one of the hCG diet

Now that you have all your supplies with you, it is time to go into the first phase of the hCG diet. This is known as the intro phase or the loading phase. For the first two days of this diet plan, you are able to eat whatever you would like. You can eat any sweet that you want, not having to worry about calories and just have fun. In fact, you should be taking in a lot of extra calories during this day so that you can prepare for the rest of the diet plan.

One of the purposes of this particular phase is that it helps to reduce temptations when you begin the second phase. But what you should really focus on is providing the body with lots of extra fat supplies so that it can make it through the rest of your hCG diet.

You should be smart about the way that you load during this phase. This can make a big difference on how good you feel when the hCG diet starts and it ensures that you are not going to get sick or not have the right nutrition. While you are allowed to eat whatever you would like, it is best to keep the focus on healthy fats rather than on the carbs and sugars. You can eat a little bit of these, but most of your meals should have as many of the healthy fats as you can find.

The good news is there are quite a few healthy fats available so you shouldn't have any issue with finding something tasty to eat for the first few days of this diet plan. Some of the options that you can choose from include nuts, salmon, and avocado because they contain a lot of healthy omega 3 fatty acids. Dairy is another good place to start because there are some healthy fats inside and any type of animal fats will work out too; so, fill up your plate with some good meat.

This is the time to break out some of those dishes that you usually keep out of your diet. This means that you should break out those cheesy chicken dishes and even the guacamole because they contain some of the fat that you need. Add some butter on top of your meals as well to really fill up. This whole phase is about getting excited for the second and the third phase of the diet; so, plan ahead of that. Also, make sure that you increase your water intake as well.

During this time, you should continue on with a good exercise program. If you already have one that is approved by a doctor, go ahead and keep going with this one as well. But if you are new to exercise or you haven't done any exercise in a long time, it is time to get started. You should pick one that is pretty light and doesn't have too much intensity so that you can build up your strength. Daily movement of some kind for a minimum of 20 minutes each day is the best option.

There are a lot of great exercises that you are able to choose from to see the results you want. Pilates, swimming, light resistance training, stretching, yoga, and brisk walking makes good choices for someone who is just getting started. Your goal with this is not really for calorie burning or fat burning, but it is more for you to build up some healthy habits. This will help you with maintaining your weight when you enter phase four of this diet plan. Plus, there are so many great benefits of exercising on your health; so, now is a great time to get started.

The first phase of the hCG diet is one of the easiest to follow, you just need to make sure that you are taking in the right types of foods. It is fine if you want to eat some carbs and sugars during this time, but the main point of this phase is to help you take in more healthy fats that can help you out when the other two phases of the hCG diet start. But with a little planning, you will be able to load up your body the right way on this diet plan and see the results that you want.

Chapter 4: Phase Two of the HCG Diet

Now it is time to move into the second phase of the hCG diet. The first phase only lasted for two days so that you can load up the body and make sure that it has the right nutrients to go through the rest of the diet. Once those two days are up, it is time to move into the second phase or the weight loss phase.

This is going to be the time period where you will see huge weight loss results. You may be able to see from one to two pounds of weight loss each day depending on how well you can stick with the diet plan and you take your hCG supplement. Let's take a look at some of the rules for following this second phase so you can see the weight loss that you desire.

First off, it is generally agreed that you should stick around 500 calories a day while on this diet plan. This is kind of a guideline though. For example, if you are someone who participates in a lot of intense exercises, it is fine to add in a bit more to help you not feel too hungry. But for most people who are lightly active or sedentary, the 500 calories will be just fine.

While this is going to seem like a very small calorie intake, you will find that it is not that bad. In fact, when you are on this diet plan and taking the hCG supplement, you may even have trouble eating just the 500 calories. These will seem like big meals to you and you will feel full and satisfied when you are done. Some people even had to be encouraged to eat more so they could provide the body with the right nutrition.

Since you will reduce the amount of calories that you consume by quite a bit, it is important that you are still providing the body with the right types of nutrients so that it can function properly. There are a few rules that you can follow when planning out some of your meals on the hCG diet. These include:

No fats: you should have gotten all the fats that you need during the loading periods earlier in phase one. But during the time you are on the hCG diet, you should not eat any extra fats. That is because the foods that have a lot of fat in them will be high in calories, making it hard to stay within your calorie allowance and feel good. It is possible to use some, but most people agree it is not worth eating 100 calories just for a small bit of oil when they could use it on other foods.

Protein: if you want to make sure that your muscles stay nice and strong on this diet plan, you need to make sure that you eat enough protein. It is recommended that you eat about a gram of protein for each kilogram of weight. Choose options that are lean, such as chicken and white fish. Dairy is usually not allowed, but if you do go with this option, choose easy options like fat-free cottage cheese or yogurt. You probably don't want to get your protein from nuts because these are going to be high in calories for the little amount you get.

Fruits and vegetables: these are going to be the biggest food group on this diet because they can provide you with a ton of great nutrients without having to worry about too many calories. These fruits and vegetables will provide you with fiber, minerals, and vitamins to make you feel great on the hCG diet. Consume them as a snack or with your protein during a meal for the best results.

A few carbs: you are allowed to have some carbs on the hCG diet, but you need to be careful with the amount. This is because carbs are often high in calories as well and you need to keep your amount down. It is best to stick with something easy like breadsticks or rice cakes. For some people, eating carbs can make them have cravings and will throw them off their goals. If this is something you deal with, just don't eat carbs.

Drinks: you are allowed to have a few different drinks on this diet. Coffee is allowed, but no added sugar, creamers, or anything else. Black tea is fine as well. But for the most part, you should only take in water. This helps you to stay hydrated and it is so important to help the metabolism stay strong. While on the hCG diet, you are not allowed to consume soda, juices, or alcohol.

How long should I do this phase?

There are a lot of different thoughts out there about how long you should stick with the second phase of the hCG diet. This part is not something that you will stick with forever, but it is a powerful phase to help you lose weight. Figuring out when you should stop this phase and move into the third phase can be the hard part.

Some experts recommend that you don't use this phase of the hCG diet more than six weeks. They believe that going much past this point with the low-calorie diet will cause the body to enter starvation mode and will ruin the results that you seek. In addition, there are some worries that if you take the hCG hormone too long, it is possible to build up an immunity to it.

Studies on the hCG diet show that it is fine to go past the six-week mark if you would like and you are still seeing results. Some people report that it wasn't until they reached the four-week mark before they saw some true momentum with their weight loss and some big changes in their body composition. Many like to go through this process for about eight weeks so that they are able to see the best results.

It is going to depend a lot on your own personal habits and how your body reacts to the hCG. Some people who need to lose a lot of weight may do better sticking with the second phase of hCG for eight weeks or more. If you are almost to the end of your weight loss goals before you get to eight weeks, it is fine to move on to the third phase of this diet plan.

Over the six to eight weeks, many of those who tried out this diet plan ended up losing one to two pounds each day, which is much more than you are able to get on other diet plans. But there are some who ended up stalling on the diet plan and falling into a plateau. Here are a few things that you can do to help overcome a plateau if you end up falling into it:

Take a look at your work: were you really that good at following the diet or did you have a lot of cheat days? If there are some improvements that you can do, it is time to make them and finish up strong.

How much water are you drinking? Going with too little or too much can sometimes cause water retention, which will show up on the scale.

Did you drink any juices, sodas, or alcohol on the diet? If you did, you should stop this immediately.

Did you take the time to exercise: exercise is so good for you, but sometimes the muscle gain that you get from it will seem like you have gained weight.

In the beginning, you're going to lose more weight. But as your body slims down, your weight loss will slow down a bit. The good news is that if you stay consistent and pay attention to your fat loss on the body, and not just your weight loss, you will see that your body is still changing on the hCG diet, even if the scale is not moving that much.

Taking the hCG hormone

Not only do you need to be careful about the foods that you are eating, and the amounts that you consume, but you need to make sure that you take your injections of the hCG hormone. This is one of the most important parts because it is responsible for helping you to speed up your metabolism and is great because it won't make you feel hungry even though you are restricting your calories.

To get started, you need to pick out the hCG that you would like to use. Make sure to get a high-quality product that has been tested and has good reviews. The injection versions are the only ones that are considered legal at this time so it is best to pick one of those since they have to meet specific guidelines. Some of the other things that you will need for this include:

An alcohol wipe
A vial that has the medication
The syringe and needle, these should be included in the package.
Some people like to have gloves to keep it sanitary.
Sharps container

There are several places where you will be able to place the hCG hormone. The first place to try is in your upper arm. To do this, uncover the arm all the way to the shoulder so you can pick out a good place. The person giving the shot should stand a little behind you while your hand is on your hip. The best place to do it is right in between the shoulder and the elbow and then shoot the hormone into the skin.

The stomach can be used as well. Uncover the stomach and look for the waist area. You will want to give the shot right below the waist but have it above the hip bone. Also look from where the body will curve at the side to about two inches from the middle of your stomach. You do want to be careful that you are not using the area that is two inches from the belly button on either side.

And you can do the injection in the thigh. You will want to have the entire leg uncovered and then look for the area that is right in between the hip and the knee. You can then go from the mid-front to the mid-side, staying on the outside part of the thigh to keep things safe.

Any of these parts will work to help you inject the hCG hormone in the right place. The important thing is to make sure that you take the right amount at the right time of the day. Each injection brand that you choose will have different rules so make sure to read the directions for the type you picked out before starting.

Some will want you to do this once a day while others will pick before each meal.

The apple day

There are sometimes when you follow this phase of the hCG diet where you will end up reaching a plateau for a few days. This is basically a period of time that lasts four days where you will not lose any inches or weight while on the diet. In most cases, the body will work through this stage as long as you keep with the diet plan and don't start to have a lot of cheat days in there. With that being said, getting stuck on a plateau for this long on the hCG diet can cause some stress and worry.

This is why an alternative has been designed that will help you to kick the body back into weight loss mode so that you are sure the plateau won't last forever. This alternative is going to be called the "Apple Day". During the apple day, the dieter is going to only be allowed to eat six apples during a 24-hour period. They can include a bit of water during the day as well, but no other foods or fluids will be allowed.

While it is tempting to just jump on an apple day whenever you don't see a ton of weight loss during the second phase, there are a few things to note. First, it is pretty normal for the body to hit a plateau and it is something that all dieters will eventually reach. But these will usually fix themselves, it is more an issue that the dieter got used to losing all that weight and becomes worried that the diet is no longer works. Make sure to check out your inches lost, and not just your weight loss so you can see all of the changes that your body is making.

If you are really worried about the plateau or it is lasting more than five days, it is fine to break it up with an apple day, but only after you have checked a few things first. First, consider if you are drinking enough water on the diet because dehydration can stop your weight loss goals. Also, check the quality of your hCG supplement. If the hCG is older than four weeks, the potency can sometimes decrease and you may need to get some new supply. And finally, check that you are getting enough sleep. If all of these things are in order and your weight loss has still stalled, it is time to add in an apple day.

So, once you have determined that it is time to start an apple day, there are a few rules to follow. Your apple day is going to start at lunch on the day that you choose and will continue until lunch on the following day. You are allowed to have up to six big apples and that is it for food that day. Any time that you feel that you are hungry, you can eat another apple. Some people only go through like four a day and that is fine, as long as you don't eat more than six.

Other than the maximum six apples and some plain water, you are not able to eat anything else. Even your water intake should be limited. You are basically allowed to drink just the amount that you need after eating the apples if you are still incredibly thirsty during the day. And always remember that you do need to take the hCG drops or injections during this day as well.

You will be surprised at the amount of weight loss that you can enjoy on that second day, mostly thanks to eliminating water in the body. And since the water will not be regained when you go back to the 500 calories from before, you will start to see more weight loss as you continue on with the diet plan.

The second phase of the hCG diet is the part that will last the longest. This part of the diet is meant to help you to lose weight quickly, usually between one and two pounds a day while you are on it, without having to feel hungry or deprived all the time. If you are able to stick with it for six to eight weeks (or a bit longer if your weight loss goals are extreme), you will be happy with the results that you see.

Chapter 5: Phase Three of the HCG Diet

Phase three is going to be like a transition phase. In phase two, you focused on restricting your calorie intake and took the hCG hormone but you are not able to stay on that kind of diet plan for the rest of your life. You also need to have some sort of transition phase between being on 500 calories a day to being back to your 1500 calories or more each day, or you are going to feel very sick. While we will talk about some of the things that you can do in the maintenance phase (also known as phase 4 in some cases), this phase is going to be all about transitioning over.

This third phase is very important to your overall success on this diet plan and it is important that you do not skip over it. Some people feel they can go right from phase two over to the maintenance phase, but this will cause some issues and could end up sabotaging all the hard work you did. The main purpose of this third phase is to help you stabilize your weight while also helping the body to adjust to normal eating habits again. If you use it in the proper way, it is also a great way for you to figure out which foods make you gain the most weight and whether or not you are dealing with food sensitivities.

Once you have reached your weight loss goal or spent about eight weeks in the second phase, it is time to move into maintenance. The point with this phase is to help ourselves return to a normal and healthy weight while maintaining it and not gaining it all back. It is very important to teach the body how to stabilize while still getting to eat a bit more than before, but always in moderation.

The biggest issue here is that when you start to add in some of the food groups to your diet again, it is easy to overdo it. Your body will crave some of those foods and so it will ask you to keep eating more. During the second phase that you just finished, you got your body used to eat a stricter diet plan and you avoided whole food groups to make sure that you got the results that you want. But once you are allowed to add some of those back into the diet, your safety zone may be gone and it can be challenging.

The important thing to remember during this stage is that you need to stay focused. Try to remember how far you came in that second phase. The good news is that this phase is supposed to last about three or four weeks. This allows you a chance to slowly add in the foods again, perhaps just a little at a time, so you won't give into temptation.

One way that you can do this is to just increase your calories first. For the first week or so, stick with only the foods that were allowed in the second phase of the hCG diet, but increase the calories a little bit at a time.

For the first few meals, this is going to be hard because your body adjusted to eating less, but if you do it a little at a time, you will adjust. As you increase the calories, make sure to check to see whether your weight is remaining steady or not.

After you have increased your calorie intake using the foods that were allowed during phase two, you can move on to the next step, which is to introduce foods that you had to take out during this diet plan. Start out slowly and remember that the goal is to never get back to what you did before, or the weight will all come back on. You may find during this stage that some of the non-hCG foods are going to trigger you to overeat; it is best to avoid these as much as possible. This will be a learning experience the whole time.

The biggest mistake that a lot of people make with the hCG diet is that they make assumptions about what they are able to eat once the diet plan is over. They assume that since all of the weight is gone, they are able to just go back to their old ways of eating and will be fine. But if you go back to the eating habits that you enjoyed before, you will just gain all of the weight back. You have to first take things slowly, the body is used to the low calories so if you leave that right away, the weight comes back. Plus, never go back to the diet plan that you enjoyed before. The hCG diet should have helped you to gain some healthier eating habits so use this to your advantage.

Always listen to your body during this stage. If you are only able to increase the calories by a little bit every few days without feeling sick, then stick with that option. If you find that eating some foods trigger you to overeat, make sure that you cut these out of your diet. Each person is going to react a bit differently to the hCG diet and getting back to a normal diet will take some time. But if you are careful and listen to the cues you get from your body, you will be just fine.

Tips to keep you on track

The transition to the maintenance phase can be one of the hardest parts of the hCG diet. You have already trained your body to go on fewer calories and with the help of the hCG hormone, you probably didn't feel that hungry or deprived either. But now that you stop using the hCG and you are bringing some foods back into the diet plan, you have to make sure that you stay on track and don't gain all of the weight back.

The first thing that you should do is to stay away from any of your trigger foods. You may have looked forward to indulging once the second phase was over, but before you dig into as many sweets as you can handle, think of how this is going to affect you. It is fine to have a little bit but consider going with a small chocolate square rather than a whole giant candy bar. If you binge on this phase too much, all that weight will just come back on.

You should also keep weighing yourself throughout this phase of the diet. You don't want to fall into denial, assuming that the weight is still off while it is creeping back on. If you get on the scale and see that the weight has gone back up, you need to do something about this right away. If you wait too long to do a weigh-in, you can gain quite a bit of the weight back and not realize it. Now you don't need to weigh each day like you did in phase two, but try to do it every few days.

As always, you should pay attention to how your body reacts when you are in this phase of the diet. You will want to start with one new food at a time and see how your body reacts to it. You may be surprised to find that you have some intolerances to some foods, sensitivities, and even some that will trigger you to overeat and gain weight. Going with one food product at a time will help you to catch some of these sensitivities early on. For example, start with some dairy products and then if the body is fine, add in some wheat products after a few days. If you notice that one of these products is causing lots of cravings, weight gain, or bloating, it is time to leave them out of the diet.

Exercise is still important even during this transition phase. Don't think that just because the main part of the diet plan is over it means that you can go back to just doing exercise on an occasional basis. You should stick with the regular exercise program that you had during the second phase of this plan, but consider picking it up a little bit more.

There are so many benefits to keeping up with a good exercise program. It will help you to keep with that healthy weight, even though you are taking in more calories now, and will be critical if you want to stay in good shape. Including physical activity on a regular basis is one of the healthy lifestyle changes that you need to adapt and continue no matter which phase of the hCG diet you are in.

Another thing that you should work on while on this diet plan is to not obsess. Some people really enjoyed how easy it was to lose weight during the second phase of the hCG diet and this weight loss can become a bit addictive. Sometimes, it is hard to convince yourself to start adding in the calories again because you like seeing all of the weight loss occur so quickly. This is a fear that a lot of people have on the hCG diet, but obsessing over this too much is just going to make you feel miserable.

You need to be reasonable with yourself. You will not be able to keep seeing the same kind of weight loss, even in the second phase, forever, and sticking with that low calorie of a diet is not healthy for too long term. But when it comes to increasing your calories, it is time to apply some of the lifestyle changes that may not make you lose more weight, but will help you to continue seeing the results that you want.

If you are worried about losing control and gaining all that weight back during the transition and the maintenance phase, it is time to make sure that your support group is in place. Talk to your doctor on a regular basis if they were there to help you out in the beginning. Join a new fitness group or find a forum online to talk to when things get stuck. These are great ways to make some new friends who can motivate you and will share your goals.

The third phase of this diet plan is all about helping you to finish off with the second phase, the phase that had you severely restrict your calories while taking the hCG hormone, and then move on to the maintenance phase where you will consume a healthy diet on a daily basis without gaining weight. It can sometimes be one of the hardest phases. You are able to add some new foods to your diet plan that were not allowed before, but you still need to be careful that you don't eat foods that will cause you to overeat or that you don't gain weight too fast. Taking things slowly is one of the best ways to succeed with this part of the diet plan.

Chapter 6: Exercising on the HCG Diet

One thing that we have not discussed yet about the hCG diet is exercising. It is important to add in some exercise to really see the results that you would like. This exercise will help you to lose weight, tone up, and get more results than just the diet and the hCG hormone can do on their own.

It is a good idea for you to exercise when you are on the hCG diet. Exercise will help you to burn more calories and see faster weight loss, and it is so important if you want to stick with a healthy lifestyle and maintain your weight loss when the hCG diet is all over. In addition, you will be able to gain all of the good health benefits that come from exercise such as fighting diabetes, fighting heart risks, and so much more.

Getting exercise on this plan

It is important for you to start being more active as soon as you are ready to get going on the hCG diet. It doesn't really matter how active you were beforehand or what shape you are in. You will just need to make some modifications and perhaps pick some easier workouts if you haven't done a regular exercise program in the past. But anyone fitness and activity level can start out their hCG diet with exercising.

If you are going on this diet plan with the help of a support team, such as your doctor or a coach, consider discussing exercise with them. Most of the time you will be able to stay with your active lifestyle throughout the hCG diet, especially if you did these intense activities before the diet plan. You do need to remember that the hCG diet is really low on calorie so working out too much can be hard since you will have trouble getting in all of the calories and the nutrition that the body needs. Unless you are used to higher intensity activities, pick something that is low impact and good for you, especially when you first get started.

The good news is that there are quite a few exercise programs that you are able to do so you can pick the one that is the best for you. You should always listen to what your body is telling you to do. For example, if you think that starting out with this diet and beginning a brand-new exercise program is going to be too hard for you, go ahead and get started with the diet plan and then implement the exercise a few weeks later when you adjust.

During this time, you should not stick with cardiovascular exercises that are really intense. When you do this, you are going to end up raising your heart rate quite a bit. This will result in the body storing all the calories that you eat into fat. Based on our ancestors who had to put a lot more effort than we need to do today, whenever our bodies sense danger (which would be the strenuous activity of cardio exercise), it will begin to preserve the calories we eat as fat.

While you are on the hCG diet, you will not want your calories to be stored as fat because that will defeat the goal of weight loss. This means that while you are on the hCG diet you need to avoid things that are really intense. You can do some exercise that gets the heart pumping a bit, like walking at a brisk pace, but you should not spend hours doing athletic training.

Picking the right time to do a workout is important as well. You should stick with about 30 minutes each day, but no more than 60 minutes. And then make sure that you get the workout done before the first meal of the day so that you can replenish the body.

You can always change up the workout that you are doing. Listen to your body for some cues on what you should be working out for that day. For example, you may enjoy going on a brisk walk for your workout most days, but if your body is worn out or you don't feel quite right on one of the days, you can try to do some relaxing yoga instead.

Add in some yoga

One of the best workouts that you are able to do on

the hCG diet that is good for the whole body is yoga. It is highly recommended because it can stretch the whole body but it won't cause harm or overexert the body. It has been shown that yoga will be able to burn through the same amount of fat as jogging without having the bad benefits for overexerting your heart.

Pick out a type of yoga that is not going to be too intense and keep the sessions short. Light yoga is plenty to help increase your blood circulation while promoting a sense of well-being and improving your own personal range of motion. You do not need to get the heart rate up that high even while doing yoga and twenty to thirty minutes is fine to get the results.

Strength training

Some people enjoy doing strength training because it helps them to get lean and strong muscles. But since you are reducing your calories so much and it is hard to get the nutrition that you need for strenuous workouts, strength training or intense resistance training are not recommended, at least when you first start out with the diet plan. In some cases, such as you have been working on strength training for years and will adjust some of your caloric needs to fit this workout, your doctor may approve you for this. But always get approval before starting.

Another thing that you have to watch out for when you work on weight training is that this is going to

143

build up your lean muscle mass. This lean muscle is going to weigh more than fat so it can make it seem like you are not losing weight when you get on the scale. If you do use this during the second phase of the hCG diet, you may want to take body measurements as well to see some of the results.

Strength training may not be the best thing for you to do during the second phase of this diet plan, but it can be great to add in when you reach phase three and the maintenance phase. For those who are just getting started, you will want to take it easy and listen to what your body tells you. Drink plenty of water during the workout as well.

Swimming

Swimming can be another choice that you can make when it comes to picking out a good workout plan on the hCG diet. This one can be safe for most people thanks to the limited impact on your joints and bones. This exercise will increase your fitness levels and can be relaxing for a lot of people. If you want a workout that will reduce your stress levels, help with a sore back, and get you out of your sedentary lifestyle, swimming is one of the best options. It will also help those who want to fight away aging or who are recovering from injuries and accidents.

If you are not used to swimming or have never used this as a workout plan, you should not spend your time doing a ton of laps all over the pool. There are often some group swimming classes, even ones for beginners that can help you to get started. Pick an activity level that is comfortable for you.

Working out is an integral part of the hCG diet. This activity is going to help you to lose weight even faster than just dieting and taking the hormone and can set you up with a new healthy lifestyle choice that will be great when you reach the transition and the maintenance phase and can add in some more foods to enjoy. You just need to be careful and always listen to your body. There are many great activities and it is always great to start with working out, but if you feel that this is too hard at the beginning, it is fine to avoid physical activity for the first few weeks and add it back in when you have adjusted to the diet plan.

Chapter 7: Maintaining the Results after the Phases Are Done

This is the part of the diet that can sometimes be the hardest, and that is why it is often known as phase 4 of the hCG diet. Reintroducing more calories and eating more food can be hard on the body. You have been restricting yourself for so long that the body is probably ready to just jump right in and eat as much food as possible. But when you are on a 500 calorie a day diet for eight weeks, there are a number of problems that can come from this. First, eating too much will make you feel sick, especially after long times with eating so few calories. Second, if you keep eating like that, all of the weight you lost will just come back.

During this fourth phase or the maintenance phase, you will be able to start introducing starches and some sugars, as well as a few more calories, back into your diet. You will want to wait until your weight has become a bit more consistent and stable. In the beginning of the hCG diet, you are going to lose quite a bit of weight from the hormone and the restricted calories. But over time, the weight loss will start to become more consistent. When you start to see this happening, it is time to enter into the fourth phase.

146

You should start out slowly, reintroducing just a few things at a time and slowly increasing how many calories that you are consuming each day. For example, adding an extra serving of bread for dinner for a few days and then maybe a dessert few days later will be good place to start. You should never go on a binge at the end of this diet plan or your body will not be happy. Always watch your body and see how it reacts to these items when you start to put them back in the diet.

One thing that you should remember is that while you did eat some of these items before, your body is going to see them as foreign and it may react to them a bit differently than it did in the past. You have to give the body some time to figure out how to burn them off. But by the time you are done with this last phase, you will have the knowledge of knowing how to eat the right foods that are good for your body, in the right amounts, while still losing weight.

You should have gained a lot of knowledge during this time as well. For example, even though you only gave up sugar for a few months, when you come back to it you may be surprised at how yucky you find its taste. You may prefer to have fruits and vegetables and other healthy snacks rather than reaching for the soda or the candy because those healthier foods now taste better. This may have been something that was impossible to do in the beginning, but thanks to the hCG diet, you have made your body crave healthier foods, rather than the high-calorie junk that you used to eat before.

One of the most important things that you will need to do during this last phase of the hCG diet is to maintain your weight, and this can be harder than it sounds. If you go into this phase, ready to eat as much food as you can and binging, or you go back to the eating habits that you had before, you will just gain all of that weight back and all the hard work that you put into the diet plan will be for nothing.

So, while you are on the hCG diet, you need to make sure that you are making some lifestyle changes in the process. This is the only way that you will see results that last. The eating plan on the hCG diet and afterward, are all about offering you a healthier way to eat, and should not be just a quick fix to help you lose weight as quickly as possible. Yes, you are going to be able to lose a lot of weight in a short amount of time, but this should be used as a way to kickstart a healthier lifestyle, not a way to just lose weight and then fall back into the same patterns as before.

There are a few things that you can do that will help you to keep your weight off and still stay healthy even after you are done with the hCG diet. First, you need to make sure that you stick with foods that are locally grown and fresh. These are less likely to have the added bad nutrients and calories that you should be avoiding. You can also stick with some meals that are pretty simple to make, such as soups, fresh vegetables, and whole grains. Cutting off the fat from the meat you eat can shave off some of the calories while helping you to still get all the good protein and other nutrients that the body needs.

If you are worried about maintaining your weight when you are all done with the hCG diet, you may want to consider finding a good eating plan that you can stick with. You will not be able to stick with the hCG diet past the first three phases because long term low calorie diets can be hard on your health. But there are a lot of good meal plans that you can pick from that will complement the hCG diet and can help you to keep the weight off.

In many cases, this last phase of the hCG diet is going to be one of the hardest ones to follow. You have to be able to maintain the weight loss that you have received from the other three phases, and this is hard when it is time to start adding some of those old favorite foods back into the mix. But with some pre-planning and some healthy lifestyle changes, you will be able to make it happen.

Conclusion

Thanks for making it through to the end of this book, let's hope it was informative and able to provide you with all of the tools you need to achieve your goals whatever they may be.

The next step is to get started on the hCG diet. This diet plan is unlike any others. While some of the other options on the market are hard to follow and don't provide you with much in terms of weight loss, the hCG diet is different. If you are able to stick with the calorie restrictions and take your hCG hormone at the right times each day, you can lose one to two pounds each day. What other diet plan has been able to promise you this?

This guidebook has provided you with all the details that you need to get started on the hCG diet. We went over some of the basics of the hCG diet, like who can benefit from going on this diet and how to get started, before moving on to the three phases of the diet that will help you see results. For anyone who wants to lose weight quickly or improve their health before things take a turn for the worse, the hCG diet is the right one for you.

If you are tired of trying out other diet plans that are hard and never seem to produce results, it may be time to try out the hCG diet. Make sure to check out this guidebook to learn everything that you need to know to get started on this diet plan today!

Finally, if you found this book useful in any way, a review on Amazon is always appreciated!

Made in the USA
Coppell, TX
25 April 2020